lessons in taxidermy

Bee Lavender

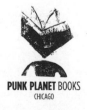

PUNK PLANET BOOKS
CHICAGO

Published by Punk Planet Books/Akashic Books
©2005 Bee Lavender

Punk Planet Books is a project of Independents' Day Media.

Cover illustration by Gabriel Liston
Book design by Pirate Signal International

The lyrics, "Our lives shall not be sweated from birth until life closes / Hearts starve as well as bodies; give us bread, but give us roses," which appear on page 133, are from the song "Bread and Roses" by James Oppenheim, words, and Martha Coleman, music (*Sing Out!*, Volume 25, 1976).

The lyrics, "All the agonies you suffer / You can end with one good whack / Stiffen up, you orn'ry duffer / And dump the bosses off your back!" which appear on page 135, are from the song "Dump the Bosses off Your Back" by Utah Phillips.

ISBN-13: 978-1888451-79-5
ISBN-10: 1-888451-79-3
Library of Congress Control Number: 2004115618
First printing
Printed in Canada

Punk Planet Books
4229 N. Honore
Chicago, IL 60613
books@punkplanet.com
www.punkplanetbooks.com

Akashic Books
PO Box 1456
New York, NY 10009
Akashic7@aol.com
www.akashicbooks.com

for my mother

AUTHOR'S NOTE

Out of respect for the privacy of the people who appear in these pages, certain names and identifying details have been changed or withheld.

home

The wind was blowing across the Puget Sound and into Seattle, bringing with it a tang of salt in the air. I stood in the middle of a neglected garden and inhaled the odor of my childhood, thousands of languorous days and nights next to the water. Growing up, I played on the rocky beaches that hug the divide between the forests and the water, with mountains towering above.

It was midnight and everyone in the house was asleep, but I felt uneasy. Something off-kilter was keeping me awake; a physical sense of apprehension was building in my stomach. I walked down the front steps to the street, skirting the snails that crawl out of the rock wall at night, the stones of the stairs shifting under my feet. One part of me attended to the shadows in alleys, but there was nothing to fear there. Nobody would bother me; nobody would even look twice as I trudged along.

I walked four blocks over a steep hill to a bluff that stands
high above industrial flats, a glittering grid of docks and ware-
houses far below. Standing on a patch of wet grass I looked west
across the inlet toward the outline of the Kitsap Peninsula illu-
minated by the moonlight, about six miles away in geographical
terms but requiring either a long ferry ride or a hundred-mile
drive around the inlets. The peninsula is more populated now,
but when I lived there it was mostly forest with a few small towns
and military installations tucked away behind stands of trees. It
was too dark to see the Olympic mountain range beyond.

I am descended from one of the first pioneer families that
homesteaded land on the peninsula, and most of my relatives still
live within thirty miles of the original farm. They work in the
shipyard, on the ferries, in gas stations, or in wrecking yards. A
few of my cousins have joined the military and traveled the world
but they almost always move home again when their tour of duty
is over. Growing up in our rural enclave, I was always jealous of
their certainty, wounded by their casual convictions. My cousins
had advantages; they could work with their hands, walk the fields,
move forward with an easy familiarity. They knew exactly where
they belonged, and I watched them with a hungry desperation. We
grew up in the same place, we were connected by blood and
history, but I was different, separate, strange. I looked across the
water and sighed. My stomach did not feel better and I turned to
walk back home.

Quietly wandering through the house, ignoring the pain, I
touched the yellow Formica table in the kitchen for scratches,
then checked that my old chipped bowls and plates were stacked
correctly, with various colors alternating. The room is host to
dozens of pictures of strangers' children, small boys of a pre-

vious century smiling as they go on pony rides or pose in long forgotten studios, and I stopped at each one, adjusting the frame, wiping dust off the glass. There are no pictures of my family on the walls; the photographs of my own children are tucked away, hundreds of images hidden in boxes, as though it would be unseemly to boast about my great luck in knowing them. Instead there are these other children, rescued from rummage sales and piles of garbage, children presumably once loved by their own mothers but later discarded by uncaring hands. In the hallway I paused to straighten a panoramic print of an army troop standing in orderly rows, ready to depart for the trenches of World War I.

The feeling in my stomach was getting worse. I brushed my teeth, holding the edge of the sink, each upward thrust of the toothbrush a chore. Looking in the mirror I saw a pale face covered with heavy makeup; and then, as though my childhood double vision had been restored, I saw one face superimposed over another, the mask of daily life sliding out of focus as the dreaded ugliness of an earlier time came into view. The face in the mirror had a frowning mouth covered in dark red lipstick to conceal lips that are losing pigment. There were lines across a forehead, but not from age—the lines were there when I was seven, nine, thirteen, twenty, frowning in concentration. Beads of sweat melted the makeup applied to cover ancient facts: scars, or the risk of additional scars. The eyes looking back at me from the mirror were haunted, terrified, no matter what the grown-up self wanted to believe. I saw everything: the past and the present, the solutions and sorrow. I wanted to put my fist through the image in that mirror. Instead I turned away, looked down, found the hairbrush.

It can take twenty minutes to untangle my long unruly hair and sometimes I just tie it in a knot on top of my head. But the party I had attended earlier that night had been in a club, with people smoking and laughing; it was imperative to remove the stench of smoke from my hair. Sitting on the edge of the bathtub I separated sections, lifted a hand, and started to yank a wooden brush through the bramble.

At that precise moment I was undone by a formidable, ghastly pain radiating outward from the guts protected by my rib cage. This was not indigestion, food poisoning, or a virus; there was something seriously wrong. I gasped and doubled over, dropping the brush. No, this was impossible. It could not be happening.

I didn't want to disturb my sleeping family; I didn't want to cause any kind of scene. I'm tough, capable of withstanding any sort of crisis. I do not need anyone to look after me, take care of me, cosset and soothe. The people who live in this house are my companions, not my caretakers.

Creeping into the bedroom, I pulled the shade against the light from a neighbor's television shining through plate glass windows, lying down on top of the covers fully dressed, trying not to shift or twitch, but the pain intensified. After an hour of tormented stillness I stood up, moving unsteadily, and walked to the bathroom. I sat on the floor and pressed my forehead against the green tiled wall. Then the vomiting began.

The pain across my rib cage turned into a firestorm so overpowering I could barely breathe. It hurt to lie down. It hurt to sit up. Wiping my mouth with a washcloth, I wanted my mother, wanted to be a little child again, safe in her arms, face pressed against a strong shoulder.

I counted to 100, said the alphabet backwards, and when that did not work tried to think of something else. I wanted to be somewhere else, be someone else. I cannot abide getting sick, the visceral experience of illness: vomit, pus, blood, the grinding reality of infection, inflammation, incapacity.

When the nausea subsided, I paced through the house, trying to look at all of my possessions and take an account of tasks and chores to do, my thoughts jumbled and inconsequential. The pine tree in the front yard needed pruning. The desk should be shifted to the other wall. I forced myself to think of these things, to think of anything except my stomach.

Pausing in the middle room I knelt in front of a shelf filled with children's books from the '50s and '60s, salvaged from libraries as they were discarded, with titles like *The True Book of Numbers, The Boys' Book of Magnetism, Look at Your Eyes,* and *A Trip to the Hospital.*

Under the bookshelf, in a haphazard stack covered with thick dust, I found an old illustrated medical dictionary with a blue cloth cover. My body shuddered with the effort of remaining in one position as I turned the pages, one after the other, the gleaming, shiny paper falling softly, until I found the chapter pertinent to my current crisis. Leaning forward, one hand against my midsection and the other splayed against the wood floor, I stared at artists' renderings of organs, muscles, ligaments, minutiae.

Still on my knees I stared around the room, trying to ignore the burgeoning awfulness in my midriff, trying to think of anything other than what might be happening inside my body. Looming in the corner is an old wooden scientific cabinet, standing over eight feet high with a glass door. Looking up at it I saw some of my collections—a pickled shark and taxidermy antlers, dozens of gruesome dental prosthetic devices, rudimentary hearing aids, glass eyes, ashtrays from old nightclubs and casinos, delicate porcelain teacups, decorative cake plates, old cameras, transistor radios, and mementos from the 1962 Seattle World's Fair. The bottom shelf is crammed with boxes of undeveloped film, stacks of family pictures, old journals, and the *E.T.* scrapbook I kept as a child.

The cabinet contains articles of proof: I am a collector, a crank, most commonly described as quirky. There are countless pieces of ephemera to prove that I have a good life now and had a happy childhood, secure and confident in the love of my family. There were difficult challenges but also glass slippers and games, elaborate costumes and expeditions, an entire extended childhood that dragged on for years after all the other kids moved into a ramshackle adulthood. Or, to say it differently: I achieved a desolate, mutable maturity too soon, and smothered inconvenient and unpleasant facts about my past with the obsessive acquisition of objects and a compulsive need to put everything in order.

Either way, it didn't matter. Disease—the opposite of ease, the abasement of vigor—takes everything away in an instant. Life can go from brilliant to agonizing with no intermediate step. Accomplishments are meaningless, every prideful thought is a void. Nothing matters except the immediate moment, the neural message that life is negative: *nought*.

Staring at the cabinet, I wanted to rail, shout, scream, to protest the inescapable and entirely wrong feeling that was now the center of my existence. It was unfair, unjust, and I wanted to kick my feet against the floor, roll around in a historic tantrum, but instead stood up and started walking again.

Hours of pacing were interrupted by more vomiting, my body was convulsing with agony. My perspective on pain as an adult is flawed, imperfect, tendered by responsibility to other people. I do not want to be a burden, require care, distract anyone from the work of daily life. I do not want people to worry about me, or see the look on a friend's face when they realize the significance of a story I present as amusing. But more than anything, I do not want to be sick.

I have faced extreme physical pain, generally without protesting in any way. There was no other choice; the first nineteen years of my life were a solid, unrelieved welt of disease. Since infancy I have been able to separate my brain from my body and simply rise above it, like a magician performing an old-fashioned parlor trick, or a trained freak in a sideshow.

I stretched out on the wooden floor of the dining room, turned on my side, and pressed a pillow against my belly. Moonlight glinted on the oak floors and the pain battered against my ribs. I closed my eyes and summoned those old skills. I thought about traveling.

Walking through the streets of Florence, my friend Gabriel kept offering the La Specola museum as a potential destination. I wasn't paying too much attention, figuring there wasn't anything in the city that I needed to go out of my way to witness after the stellar experience of Machiavelli, Michelangelo, Fermi, and Marconi, all snug together next to Dante's empty tomb at Santa Croce.

"What is La Specola?"

"You know that book you have at home, about the taxidermy museum with the anatomical figures?" he asked.

"What about it?"

He shook his head. "Bee, that museum is *here*." He pointed at the ground.

"Really? Do we have time?"

Gabriel pursed his lips and looked at his watch, then pulled a train schedule out of his canvas satchel. He calculated that we could go if we hurried.

The building was quiet and empty of any other patrons. There were rooms full of plants, sea creatures, insects, hives; then leopards, jaguar, puma, male and female and infant lions, and gazelles. There was a case with deerlike creatures posed in a "natural" family group, gazing about, raising up on back legs to nibble on plants, the floor of the case covered in round brown pebbles. On the white wall of the case there was a photograph of a Saharan scene, a picture of trees and a river to provide a sense of the environment the specimens were taken from.

The floor of the hall was red tile in a crosshatch pattern, the display cases old and made of a dark, varnished wood, the glass slightly warped. One wall of cases started with cats of all kinds, but the lions and others faded away into sea lions, then bears lined up on shelves. I couldn't tell if they were meant to be baby bears or fully grown; there were varieties I'd never seen and the cards didn't help me figure out which might have been native to the forested land where I grew up.

The hallway veered into a room full of animal trophies, heads on the wall, furniture made from skins, a hollow elephant leg, and massive skulls. There was a zebra staring out from a corner cabinet, seams and stitching shabby from years of decay, followed by whales, belugas, and small dolphins.

We moved on to a room of more deer, elk, horned sheep, llamas, then monkeys of all sorts. Recorded organ music wafted in from the next room. Gabriel stepped up next to the other displays and looked at himself in a mirror. I took a picture of Gabriel in his suspenders, long-sleeved shirt, and old workpants, mixed in with the other elements. I rarely allow myself to be photographed but when I developed the film, I saw the camera had caught me in the mirror, sequined skirt glinting in contrast to the shadowy cabinet.

Just past the sharks I could see the first room of human specimens. I hurried past vague objects in jars—snakes, various strange looking fish, round, long, fat, thin, vibrantly colored or drab and muddy, big, small, crazy fins, teeth, no teeth.

I walked into the room with full-scale wax models of humans. The signs at the entrance explained that the models were made to facilitate biology instruction, since cadavers were hard to find and storage was a challenge in the eighteenth century. Fourteen-hundred wax anatomical sculptures were eventually collected and displayed in 550 cases taking up nine rooms of La Specola. The rooms had dark green curtains and the bottoms of the cases were painted to match, with a decorative green vase in each corner.

One set of cases offered hearts inside women cut open to reveal the contents of their chest cavities, heads turned slightly, hair trailing down. A woman in a glass case had long, braided hair, hands draped at her side in submission, pubic hair curling, her body open from mons to clavicle with organs draped across her chest. Another woman had her hand up, playing idly with her hair as intestines spilled out of her abdomen, her expression pensive. The third woman seemed to be in ecstasy as the deeper organs of her torso burst from the delicately rendered model.

The exhibits were mesmerizing and I moved from case to case, staring at familiar structures. Walking forward I saw details of the vertebrae, connections of the torso, the rib cage. Then the subcutaneous and deep muscles, intestines, kidneys, gallbladder, and pancreas. There was a torso of a young man with a face that looked resigned yet patrician; the note on the case said this figure had been made as a résumé to request a job.

I stopped in front of a case with a woman's head adorned with curly brown hair, cheeks detailed and lustrous, the skin of her throat rolled up to reveal the architecture of the neck, the thyroid prominent and obviously important.

Gabriel stopped with me to sketch the wax figure. I leaned close and whispered, "My first tumor, when discovered, was three times as large as the thyroid it was suckling. The doctors said that they would need to amputate my voice box. They said the cancer was terminal, a rare variety, that I would live perhaps six months."

Gabriel smiled vaguely and moved on to another case full of faces, half faces, the anatomy of eyes and ears, figures showing how tendons and muscles and arteries are entwined. There were babies, then baby eyes, then eyes of all kinds dissected and in rows.

I put my head close to the wax eyes, trying to see how the muscles connect.

I was born with profound double vision and saw everything with one eye fixed straight ahead, the other wandering, my brain calculating distances but never quite knowing where I stood in reference to my surroundings. I wanted to be a normal girl, with regular skin and ordinary clothes, commonplace hobbies and predictable friends. Before the doctors noticed my eyes, I taught myself to read by scanning two lines at once; taught myself how to ride a bicycle, how to walk on balance beams, how to twirl a baton and send it flying into the sky and then catch it again when it came back down. The doctors surgically repaired the double vision, trying to make me normal, but it took years to regain my balance.

The museum was drafty, and my old, broken bones throbbed. I shivered, shoved my hands in the pockets of my coat, and walked into another room to see little babies curled up in waxen wombs, hands folded across tummies, their faces perfectly formed and rather Napoleonic. The models were accurate in detail from the tiniest fetus to the largest infant. The growth of the uterus was displayed with remarkable acuity—surprising for a time when most scientists believed in homunculus, the theory that a child is pre-constituted in sperm—and I stopped to take notes. The babies were split open to show their internal systems, their expressions placid. Gabriel started to sketch one of the infants.

A wall of cases had sections of women, ribs to below hips, legs spread. One had twins ready to birth. Every model had pubic hair. One showed a head descending and a relatively accurate anatomy of the womb. The clitoris, labia minor and majora, and rectum were all presented in detail. The cervical opening was shown expanding, the head of the infant descending, the mons swelling during the descent. The model showed how the internal organs are displaced to accommodate the growth of the uterus.

One reclining female wearing pearls had two long braids. She stared out at me with brown eyes, her lips slightly open, looking pained and saddened, as though she needed to tell me something. She could be dismantled layer by layer down to the uterus.

When I was in the hospital waiting to give birth to my daughter, I wandered through the halls for hours and eventually found a private entrance to the teaching wing. I ignored the signs warning that no patients were allowed to enter the area and opened the door. Moving slowly, I looked at cases filled with medical specimens. The contents of those jars were extracted from real people; tumors and oddities left on display to assist and titillate medical students.

Before that moment I had never considered the fate of my own lost body parts, never thought they would be so indecently displayed. It wasn't until that slow walk in the dark hospital hallway, waiting for medical technology to trick my body into giving birth too early—parents and friends convinced I would die in the process—that I understood my own value as a specimen and experiment.

I did not want these memories, did not want to see myself as a piece of medical history. Walking further into La Specola, I stopped in front of a series of small macabre waxen tableaux. *The Triumph of Time* showed a fallen city. There were dead babies in stages of decay, fallen women still clothed, green with rot, skeletons, half decomposed people, and an angel, perhaps Michael. Rats were nibbling at intestines. In *The Pestilence* there was a mass of dead people, the live dragging bodies to piles, men, women, a grandmother, baby, and dog all dead, a confused infant clutching the skirt of his dead mother. *The Corruption of the Flesh* showed the Madonna surveying the scene from a rooftop, sadly staring at the bodies strewn about, half eaten, a man in front with his belly distended, a rat opening it, a dead baby lying beside.

Standing in the center of the museum I looked around at the profusion of objects, case after case filled with detailed renderings of all manner of suffering. I could hear a telephone ringing and a cat mewing outside and a clock ticking somewhere nearby. I wanted to go home.

fighting

At dawn, I lurched to the living room and attempted to find a diagnosis via the Internet. According to various sites, the symptoms were either inconsequential or life-threatening. When the thought *there is no hope* crossed my mind, I picked up the phone and called a medical advice line. Before I managed to describe the whole problem, the nurse interrupted to tell me I needed to be seen immediately.

I shook Byron awake and whispered, "I need to go to the hospital."

He sat up quickly, rubbing his eyes, and asked, "What happened?"

"I feel really ill in my stomach."

He reached for my hand. "What did you eat? What is happening?"

I shook my head.

He was startled; he knows that I've never asked to be taken to the emergency room. He rushed to wake our little boy and helped him shrug into his standard outfit: slacks, a long button-down shirt, and a blazer. They gathered books, paper, and colored pencils for the trip. My daughter is a teenager and had a friend staying over. They were asleep downstairs and could stay home alone, so Byron left a note on the table. We climbed into my old Volvo and, as Byron drove down the hill to the hospital, I muttered, "If they offer, I'm going to say, *Sign me up for surgery*."

He laughed and replied, "I'll remember you said that."

I gave the person at the desk my insurance information and then sat sideways on a chair in the emergency room in deep and unrelenting misery, dry heaves rippling up my esophagus, for several hours. The television in the lobby was showing the Tom Hanks movie *The Money Pit*. I closed my eyes against what may be the least funny movie I have ever had the misfortune to watch.

Every thirty minutes or so I stumbled to the public rest room and spat bile into the toilet, convinced I would pick up an infection if I so much as touched the light switch. My body still harbors traces of hepatitis acquired during a hospital stay more than twenty years ago, still bears the scars of staph infections that settled in the crevices of new incisions. I held a wadded paper towel in my hand to push the lever and flush away the fluid that had trickled out of my mouth.

I wanted to lie down on the beige, speckled floor of the hallway, but cautiously walked back to my chair, one hand held out for balance, near but not quite touching the wall.

Byron patted my arm tentatively, leaned down, and tried to make eye contact. I turned my face away, and he said, "This is really much more serious than you are letting on, isn't it?"

I nodded but kept my eyes on the aquarium on the opposite wall, watching the blue and yellow fish languidly trail through a green plastic castle.

"Please go tell them," he urged, but I shook my head no. "If you don't, I will."

"I can wait my turn," I replied, but he stood up and walked to the desk to ask the nurse to take me out of the lobby. There were no rooms available; the triage nurse was busy, the supply of people with heart conditions and nail-gun injuries was plentiful.

He kept going back to repeat the request, with the same results. Each time he sat down he urged me to make a scene. He whispered, "You need to cry or they won't understand that you are really ill. You need to make a big scene, and then you'll be pushed ahead in the queue."

I shook my head. No, I would not cry; not in a hospital, not in front of strangers.

When I was five years old my uncle Anton married a girl with permed blond hair and green eyes. The church party broke up quickly, all the presents loaded into a truck, the teenage bride and groom making out in front of the car my father and some of the other grown-ups had decorated with shaving cream and tin cans tied with string.

Back at the farm where my mother grew up, the real party started, with just our family and the neighbors and a few friends of the teenage married couple. The uncles stacked cases of Budweiser on the back porch. Grandma cooked a big dinner of macaroni noodles and tomato sauce with crumbled hamburger, store-bought greasy whole chickens, and packages of flaky, pull-apart rolls.

My mother brought plates of deviled eggs, stored in our trunk during the wedding, and she stood in the kitchen laughing and talking to her sisters as she mixed up tuna to spread on tiny pieces of sliced rye bread. My mother was wearing a green velvet dress with puffy sleeves. She was twenty-three years old, lovely and kind; she looked like the relatives from northern Finland, dark-haired blue-eyed people with high cheekbones. I leaned against her legs, rubbing my face against the softness of her skirt.

The cousins played in the back room and the grown-ups sat around the house, smoking and drinking and cracking jokes at the new couple's expense. We ate off paper plates, the plain red tomato sauce seeping through, bits of food dropping off for the dogs. People started going home, the great-aunts first, with their assorted kids and grandkids, then the teenage friends— they had other parties to go to that night. It was mainly family in the house. My mother told me to lie down on the couch, then tucked a crocheted brown and red afghan around me.

I snuggled with my little white dog, our faces resting on the flat silk pillow stitched to commemorate a stranger's trip to a foreign port. The dog had been rescued by Anton, who found him hiding in a pile of tires behind a gas station, his small body covered in cigarette burns. When the puppy first came to the farm he was afraid of people; he quaked and peed all over the hallway the first time he saw me. But I picked him up and held him close and soon we were inseparable. Anton named him Casper; a name that resonated with glamour in my young mind.

Casper became my best friend and defender, a tiny mutt smaller than a loaf of Wonder Bread, snarling at anyone who seemed to pose a threat. I fell asleep listening to my mother and her brothers and sisters, Grandma and Grandpa, and assorted husbands and wives all together, all laughing.

I woke up to the sound of glass breaking, voices raised in anger. I sat up and hugged my little dog closer, confused. My mother ran past, coming from the bathroom with towels, and said sharply, "Put on your shoes."

Had I done something wrong? What was happening? I reached down for my shiny black shoes. I slipped a small foot into one and was pushing the strap through the buckle when a roar and a chorus of screams made me look up, just as my uncle, the groom, came running straight at me, face red and mouth cracked open, eyes maniacal.

His brother was behind him, tattooed arm reaching forward to grab his shirt, and Grandpa was there too, his hand on Anton's belt. Anton screamed and it was a conquered warrior's howl, a victim's shriek, the sound of a sick and dying animal cornered and fighting back.

My uncle and grandfather leapt forward at the same time, tackling Anton, and the three bodies hurtled through the air, sliding across the coffee table in front of me, pieces of their errant bodies connecting with my knees, arm, head. They slid across the coffee table, knocking over lamps, and landed in a heap next to the front door. My little dog jumped into the fray, biting at whichever piece of flesh he could reach.

Someone grabbed me, yanked me off the couch, and it seemed like I was flying through the rooms, carried aloft like lumber, one shoe dangling, the other lost in the fray of fighting men, grunting and pummeling each other. I wailed, "No, no, my puppy!"

But whoever was carrying me ignored my yells and ran away from the fight, past the remains of supper on the big oak table, through a kitchen spattered with blood and broken glass, across the dark porch and outside. I could smell whiskey and beer and then I was standing with no coat in the yard, next to the picnic table and the sandbox, the silver-dollar plants, the willow tree, and the bride.

She was crying, and in the dim light from the nearby chicken coop I could see mascara streaming down her face and neck, making smudges on her white dress. We were alone, the rest of the family was inside; we could hear them yelling, dogs barking, but we had been set aside, sent into the exile of the yard. The foot with no shoe was wet from the dew on the grass and I could see stars and a sliver of a moon above the orchard. The bride cried and cried and I patted her arm. "It's OK," I said, "this doesn't happen very often."

Most of the family lived near the farm, but our house was on the other side of the peninsula, in a neighborhood that consisted of a few short streets bordered on three sides by a forest and on the fourth by an abandoned municipal dump. Each family had built their own house as part of a low-income government program, children holding hammers or climbing through the wooden shells of the walls before the sheetrock was delivered. The new house was the most beautiful thing I had ever seen, painted dark green like the forest. My parents had built it, I had helped, and I was bursting with pride the day we moved in. I walked through our new home barefoot, toes curling in the brown shag carpeting, then ran and slid across the yellow and brown linoleum in the kitchen.

The children of the neighborhood made paths in and out of the remnants of the forest closest to our homes. We had clearings and we had hollowed logs; there were tiny winding trails and some bigger tracks our dads made for dirt bikes.

One day I was in the woods across from my house, a tangled mass of blackberry bushes and salal and wild rhododendrons, evergreens shading our special places. We were playing a game where the girls were the pioneers in wagons, trudging across the deserts and barren plains we had seen on television Westerns. It didn't occur to me then to wonder how the pioneers who went all the way west, to the Northwest—the very furthest tip of the United States before it drops into the ocean, large tracts covered in a dense, mottled, cold, impenetrable rain forest—had managed their move. It seems like the barren plains, though barren, would have at least been easier to walk across.

Todd was the ox, tied up with a jump rope, pulling our weary pioneer wagon as we sang songs and worried about ambush. "Faster, oxen," I called to him, tapping his bottom with the wooden handle of the rope. The other girls giggled and Todd said it would take more than that to make him go faster.

I tapped his bottom harder, and he stared at me with his cold eyes, then challenged, "Is that all you can do?"

I tapped again, harder. He laughed at me and the girls giggled. "How about this?" I asked, and hit even harder. He kept laughing. I raised my arm above the soft bottom he was wiggling at me, daring me, and brought the wooden handle down with a *thwack*.

Suddenly the oxen reared up, ropes swinging in an arc, and then he wasn't a pretend animal anymore but a real one, shoving me to the ground, pinning me, hitting and scratching as I pushed and writhed and tried to get away. The red-headed girls had stopped giggling and were standing there with their mouths open, and then they ran away—not to get help, but to hide behind their high fence. I shoved at Todd above me, but I was shocked and he was a solid boy.

We rolled in the dirt and then he had his hands on my ears, on my pretty new earrings, and he clutched and yanked as hard as he could; his face was close to mine and I could feel my ear lobe tear and I started to cry and then his mouth was on my cheek, his teeth digging in, ripping the skin, the skin of my face and my ear, and I screamed and pushed and knocked him away, running for home without looking back.

I had blood on my face, blood on my neck; the earring had been ripped all the way through the lobe, leaving me not with a tiny piercing but with a large, jagged hole. My mother asked me what happened and wiped off the blood, but I sobbed. My nose and mouth filled with mucous and I started to hiccup and I couldn't say much except, "Todd hurt me."

There was a knock at the door. My mother went to answer, and I could hear the voice of Todd's mother. I ran to the pantry and hid in the very lowest cupboard, pulled the hollow sliding door shut behind me, cowering in the dark with my hands over my ears so I would not hear the conversation.

After Todd's mother left, my mother slid the pantry door open. "Come out," she said, and she didn't sound happy.

"Next time," she said, "you have to hit back."

In my family, women hit back. Sometimes they hit first. Usually not in a provocative way, not to start a fight, but in the middle of a fight, raging over some enormous transgression. It is easy to break the rules when you live not only in poverty, but in the lowest dregs of working poverty: too poor to feed your family but not poor enough to receive government benefits; a family living on a salary earned delivering newspapers or part-time work in the forest. Everyone worked too much for too little, and sometimes there would be a huge argument over something the men bought— probably a model car, a magazine, tickets to a movie, a special treat—and how that money should have gone toward a loaf of bread.

If a fight started in the car, it usually ended with the man dropped off on the side of the road, kicked out to walk home or bum a ride off a stranger. Sometimes someone would raise a hand and hit. Then they would fall on each other, stand up, fall back, do-si-do around the room in a dance of violence while I sat and watched Westerns on television.

Nobody hit me, not even as a measure of discipline. My cousins were cuffed routinely, someone was always threatening to cut a switch; smacks fell down like rain. I was told to defend myself whenever necessary, but I was protected from the adults because my mother would not let anyone touch me, and because I was a bleeder.

My nosebleeds were frequent and copious. I could soak a towel or fill the sink basin just from riding in a car or reading too long or falling asleep in an awkward position. If I felt sad I coughed up blood. I was usually sick, curled up with a blanket and an infected organ, ear, throat, taking medication and recuperating perpetually, watching television and reading books.

I saw fights between my cousin Louisa, a teenager still, with short hair and David Bowie T-shirts, and her husband. His name was Casey and he drove a VW van and wore purple high-top sneakers with plaid bell-bottoms. They used the baby's diaper bag to hide their stash of drugs. I know that when they broke up, someone hit someone else, and my cousin's eardrum was punc-

tured, but it was never clear to me why Casey was the bad guy. He
always seemed so nice. Louisa was one of my favorite people, but
one day on the way to see Laser Pink Floyd in Seattle, she wouldn't
stop kicking one of her sisters in the car. They drove into the ditch
and ended up pummeling each other in the middle of a busy road.

It was understood, though never debated, that the habitual,
reflexive violence was an expression of strength; we were not
abused but merely querulous. We were the strong ones, the victo-
rious, and women were to be honored for their ability to fight.
The aunts whispered about a neighbor named Linda who had
married a man with a moustache and mean eyes. He hit her and
she just put her hands across her eyes, crying.

Linda came over to drink coffee with bruises on her arms,
black eyes, and a big pregnant belly. My aunts said that if she
couldn't protect herself she should leave, or failing that, kill him;
they nodded and agreed that they would never let a man get away
with that shit. When Linda's baby was still in diapers, she tried to
leave, but the man broke down the door and beat her up, left her
bleeding on the floor, took his son and disappeared forever.

Some fights were so legendary and discussed so often, it was
easy to imagine you had witnessed them even if you weren't born
when the event occurred.

My Aunt Signe had a wretched husband, the worst kind of
bad imaginable. He was a drunken thief named Willy, a mess of a
person who once went out drinking and driving on a Sunday
afternoon and ran over several people walking to church. Signe
had a good job as a secretary in the naval shipyard, and one day in
the middle of an argument Willy swept up all of her work clothes
and took them outside. He threw the clothes in the muddy
driveway and then drove back and forth over them with his car.

When he came back inside he was laughing and he picked up a bottle of whiskey, raising it to his lips for a drink. She smacked that bottle into his mouth, shattering teeth and glass, bone and blood and whiskey spilling forward across the kitchen table as he screamed.

Another time they had a fight about dog food and he hit her and she grabbed a knife and chased him out of the house. Willy went down the driveway and she got in her station wagon and knocked him down and drove over him, grinding him into the mud and gravel, like he had driven over her beige pantsuits, permanent-press skirts, blouses with ruffled collars.

It didn't kill him; we believed he was too wicked to die. Once when he hobbled by, stinking of whiskey and oil, a cousin whispered, "Too bad she didn't use the truck."

In a different kind of story the neighborhood would be redeemed. The children would grow up together, learning important lessons, tempered by love and kindness and decency. We would remember our childhood as difficult because we were poor and often lonely, but we had the green, damp forest and the gray sky delivering bountiful rain, and we had each other: good friends.

But this is not that story. In the real story I was diagnosed with cancer.

In January of 1983, my twelfth birthday was celebrated in the children's ward of a small rural hospital with floral deliveries, dozens of helium balloons, and boxes of candy lining the window. The doctors had cut through strap muscles, moved aside tendons, and found a glistening tumor—a hot solid malignancy on top of a grotesque cold liquid cyst, twining around nerves and smothering my thyroid. After a preliminary culture of the tissue, they carefully excavated the vocal cords, then cut out the tumor and as much of the thyroid as could be risked. They left a suction catheter in my neck, draining blood through a tube. Nurses took my temperature and held cups of water to my mouth, telling me to swallow against the pain.

My uncle Anton gave me a toy donkey I named Nestor; a friend from school gave me a little lion I named Lucy. I gripped the stuffed animals with one arm; the other was splayed across a pillow, swollen and throbbing, blood smeared under the tape holding an IV in place. I stared at a mural of a farm scene painted in primary colors, with animals and a girl and a barn all somehow slightly skewed. The perspective was wrong, the duck too large compared to the horse, the fence too small for the pig.

The surgeon had short red hair and he whispered to my mother in the hallway. He said the news was *bad*, far worse than anyone had imagined.

I wanted to sleep, wanted to curl up and forget everything, but the pain was incandescent. Lying under white sheets, halfway decapitated to remove the tumor lodged in the front of my neck, I reached for the nurse call button but it slipped out of my hand and fell to the floor.

I couldn't move. I wanted my mother, but visiting hours were over and I was alone watching the searchlights sweep the sky above the naval shipyard. When she arrived the next morning, tears welled up in my eyes. She squeezed my hand, leaned over, and whispered, "Don't cry."

She didn't say more but I knew she meant, *Don't cry, because your tears will dissolve the adhesive of our armor. Don't cry, because you need to fight.*

Before the cancer, I played dangerous games at school, flung people down the hill behind the game fields, chased the boys into the blackberry thickets and wouldn't let them out. But after the surgery I wasn't allowed out at recess and I couldn't play, couldn't even stay awake half the day, and I lay dreaming on a yellow bench in the nurse's office, the hard, cold vinyl seam leaving an imprint on my face.

My mother had a purple T-shirt printed for me with puffy white letters: *Fragile*. It was a joke and we all laughed, but the shirt was also a factual account of my diminished status. I was not allowed to play outside.

Neighbor kids stopped coming over, and I was too tired to go to the woods. I walked home from the bus stop every day with a boy nobody ever played with named Tommy. He had grand mal seizures and profound brain damage, and conversations with him were a constant looping discourse; he couldn't remember the question he had just asked, or the answer just received. His mother never let him go to the forest. Soon the other children were insulting us, name-calling, throwing rocks when their jeers were ignored.

I heard every insult, but Tommy seemed oblivious, just happy to have someone to be with. I held my folders and schoolbooks clutched to my chest, pulled back my shoulders, and continued walking. When the rocks hit me, I won't pretend they didn't hurt, but I just kept moving.

Because I was so sick, I had my own television set with a remote control. I stayed in bed with my little white dog on my lap, all the dolls and stuffed animals people had brought to me in the hospital lining the shelves.

During the weekends I slept all day and watched television all night and found *Doctor Who*, a puzzling and aberrantly long

program that rarely made any sense but always included a girl
swept up in the service of the Doctor, a girl who could defend
herself and her companions and cleverly figure out the means of
escape from danger. I watched *The Avengers*, another British show,
with stylish secret agents. The male character wore a bowler hat
and had a cane concealing a knife. There was a girl who knew
martial arts and generally bested her male partner at every level of
resourcefulness; she could fight her way out of any situation,
either with her hands or her mind, while maintaining an impec-
cable and modish wardrobe.

I slept as the other children played outside, and my dreams
were of space travel, of fighting alien creatures. I stayed in my
room dreaming that I was an Avenger, a glamorous and dangerous girl spy.

One day in the lunchroom, next to the orange folding tables,
across from our carved wooden mascot killer whale, a boy walked
up to me and reached out a hand, placed his index finger in the
middle of the scar across my neck, and pushed. What could be the
point of this act? Did he want to impress the other kids eating
their square pizza slices and tater tots, sipping milk from waxy
cartons? Was it curiosity? A challenge? Or was it the primitive act
of a pack animal weeding out the sick and dying?

He shouldn't have touched me. I did not stop to think; I just
grabbed his wrist and twisted, shoved him against the wall,
brought my other hand up to his neck and squeezed until he
couldn't breathe. His eyes rolled in terror and the lunchroom fell
silent. "Don't touch me again," I said in my haggard new voice,
"or I will kill you dead."

changeling

The fact that I have never had to sit in an emergency waiting room as a sick person has always been a point of pride. In the past I always turned up at the hospital so far in crisis I skipped directly to admissions. As it turns out, this was an extremely smart strategy.

Resting on a flimsy blue plastic chair surrounded by people with an array of real and imaginary illnesses made me feel exponentially worse. There were homeless people looking for beds, kids with broken bones, people from other countries fallen ill abroad and trying to describe their health insurance to the intake staff. A toddler wanted to play on the floor with toy trucks but his mother yelled at him to be quiet. A man with a detached retina held a kitchen towel over his face. Teenage girls in the corner had a picnic set up; they were from a church youth group and they were supporting a friend with a sprained wrist. There was a woman who, when asked what she needed to be seen for, said, "Canker sores."

I noticed that the chairs were out of alignment, some in uneven rows, others yanked over next to the pay phone or the vending machines. It hurt my head to look at them so I closed my eyes.

The triage nurse called me to his office and took my temperature (normal), blood pressure (low), and asked about my symptoms. He nodded and made notes and seemed to think that the problem was within the scope of his usual routine.

I didn't know how to tell the man: Listen, I *never* cry and right now I am blinking back tears. Listen, and please understand, I am not what you think. My clothes and erect posture are misleading. I can pretend and I can make-believe, but the scars do not lie. I wanted to say: Imagine a winter day twenty years ago. There is a little girl with shaggy blond hair in a bowl cut, and she is prepped for surgery, on a gurney being wheeled through fluorescent hallways of a hospital. Imagine stops at various examination rooms, where teams of doctors wait to quiz her mother on radiation exposure, symptoms, surgical history. They do not offer new advice; they just want an opportunity to see a disease none of them have ever encountered.

But the pain had scrambled my thoughts; I could not even whisper responses to the triage questions. I had no answers, could not explain the truth to this man. I doubled over and rested my hands on my forehead and realized that I was still wearing the gaudy polyester cocktail dress from a party the night before.

A few weeks after the surgery on my neck there was a follow-up appointment. The young female doctor examined me and asked my mother to step out of the room to have a consultation in her office. They left me alone wearing a crinkly paper smock and I jumped down from the table, shoved my legs into jeans, yanked the turtleneck that covered the new scar over my head, and ran down the hall, pushing my way into the office.

My mother was frowning, her lips pressed together, fingers gripping her brown leather purse until her knuckles turned white.

The doctor blinked and politely asked me to leave.

"No. This is my body. You tell *me* what is wrong." My face felt hot, and I knew my ears had turned bright red.

The doctor looked at my mother and she nodded her consent. I sat down in a brown plush chair and looked out the window, waiting. Her office had a view of the parking lot and I watched an elderly man fastidiously help an old woman out of a dingy Ford.

The doctor used a plastic model to describe some points of the surgery, pulling shiny plastic skin away from the plastic larynx, moving layers of red muscle and purple tendon to show the thyroid. My heart was beating so loud I wasn't sure that I would be able to hear what she needed to tell us. She kept her eyes focused on the plastic model as she said, "Unfortunately, the tissue removed from her neck was cancerous."

We had been told this at the hospital, so there must be more news. I glanced at my mother. She nodded and waited for the doctor to continue.

"The local labs could not verify the variety, so we divided the tissue and sent it to labs around the country."

My mother nodded again, knuckles still white against the soft brown leather of her purse.

The doctor paused, and her voice was soft and low when she

said, "The preliminary tests indicate that we need to assume . . ."
She paused, shifted her pen on the desk, then looked up again.
"I'm sorry. We need to move forward with the assumption that
this is aggressive and terminal."

We stared at the doctor. The room was silent, eerie. I looked
up at a photograph on the wall behind her desk, a sailboat in a
harbor. She continued, "In the worst-case scenario, patients can
expect to live for six months. In the best, maybe a year."

My mother looked down at the floor, then stood up abruptly
and motioned for me to follow. She turned her back on the
doctor and said flatly, "Thank you. Have a nice day." We walked
out to the lobby to make a payment on the account. There were
still Christmas cards taped to the wall behind the receptionist's
typewriter, and tinsel attached to the edge of the high counter. My
mother pulled out her wallet and a calendar with a red plastic
cover to schedule the next appointment. Her hands were shaking
when she signed the check.

We drove across a metal bridge with rivets the size of my fist,
around a small inlet, and down Perry Avenue to the pharmacy.
My mother was silent, one hand on the wheel and the other fid-
dling with her cigarettes, lighting a new one off the glowing stub
of each one she finished. I looked out the window and saw the
ranch house where a veterinarian used to keep a lion caged on his
back porch. The lion had been gone for several years, but I
remembered his shaggy, sad face looking through the posts of the
cedar deck.

At the pharmacy, I sat down in the waiting area next to a large
display of Harlequin romances. The smell of roasted chicken
wafted in from a market next door. I sat slumped in the hard
plastic chair, staring at a display of pastel greeting cards.

My mother asked if I wanted anything: books, candy, a toy? I shook my head no. The pharmacist had a big handlebar moustache and he smiled down over the high counter. He asked how I was feeling. I replied, "Fine."

That weekend my mother took me to every bookstore on the peninsula, and then across the bridge to the next county, searching for books about kids with cancer. We stood together in one store after the next, going through each shelf in the children's sections, moving on to the health and medicine areas. Every time we found a book that seemed to address the topic, my mother read the description on the flyleaf before shoving the object back in place on the shelf. After two full days of searching, we had only found books that addressed grief and loss. There were no books about children who survived. The search ended in a mall bookstore near the Seattle airport. My mother was holding a paperback copy of the Lois Lowry novel *A Summer to Die* when she turned to me and said, "Promise me that you will grow up and write a book about a kid who lives."

I didn't think that I could keep the promise, but I nodded.

The routine of our days carried the family forward. I visited my grandparents at the farm, sat next to the woodstove, watched *The Price Is Right* on the television with my grandmother. I went to see my other grandparents; they owned the gas station where my father worked. Standing in the small office, I could smell grease and burning oil and gasoline. The gritty sand they used to clean the floors crunched underfoot and I peeled down the neck of my shirt to show how the scar was healing, then peered out through the glass window at customers waiting to pick up their cars.

My parents went back to work; they had no choice. One job

provided health insurance, the other an hourly wage, and they
needed every dollar they could earn to pay medical bills. I went to
school and sat in the quiet of the library, reading novels about the
Revolutionary War; one had a girl who dressed up like a boy so
she could go into battle. I read a biography of Marie Curie and
books about the Underground Railroad. The library had shelves
of fairy tales for younger children and I turned the pages of the
books over slowly, staring at the illustrations, imagining that the
illness was just a fairy curse. I thought that if I read enough books
I might find a secret incantation that would take away the cancer
and make me whole again.

The night my mother gave birth to me, two other babies were
born. We were the first of the New Year and the newspaper sent a
reporter to take a photograph. One of the other infants was my
cousin, and the medical staff mixed us up. We were only
changelings for a short while—our grandparents noticed that the
bald baby had been swapped for the one with a shock of black
hair—but maybe something more sinister had happened.
Everyone said that I had been an uncanny infant, with twirling
eyes and a preternatural ability to speak before I could crawl. My
mother taught me rhyming poems and my grandparents set me
on the counter at the gas station to recite them for the customers.
If I were really a fairy child, then a human child had been smug-
gled away and would stay alive forever, playing and running
through underground caverns.

Maybe the doctors were wrong; they had been before. When
I was a few weeks old, the pediatrician prescribed a special diet:
He told my mother to feed me apple juice instead of milk.
Consequently, my baby teeth were rotten, putrid yellow fangs. I

kept my lips pressed together, held both hands across my face whenever I laughed. The dentist who looked in my mouth at age three said that I would need extensive treatments to protect my adult teeth. Over the next decade I had a dozen root canals; half my teeth were capped with stainless steel, and eventually they were all extracted. It was difficult to sit still, hold my mouth open, breathe through my nose, ignore the smell of laughing gas and the whirring of the drills. I traced the murals of teddy bears with my eyes, recited nursery rhymes in my mind, or became a superhero flying above the treetops. The tooth fairy left five dollars under the pillow if I let the dentist pull my teeth without making a fuss.

A few weeks after the surgery on my neck, during a dental appointment, an X-ray revealed a shadow where there should have been bone. Something large and menacing was clawing through my jaw, demolishing molars that had not yet come to the surface, pushing fragments of tooth and bone up to the joint. The dentist frowned over the image and picked up the telephone. The surgery was too delicate for the local hospital. I was sent across the water to Seattle to have a portion of my face removed.

This, they assured me, was not a malignant growth. It was a cyst—a virulent, destructive, mystifying cyst. There was no connection between the cyst in my jaw and the cancer in my neck. How could this be? There was no answer.

There were very few facts available. They didn't know if they would go through my cheek or through my mouth; they didn't know if the surgery would kill nerves. They warned that I might drool constantly or bite my lips bloody, but that I would grow used to the loss of sensation. After the surgery, my mouth would be hard-wired shut, with jagged metal spikes and wires connecting all the teeth. My jawbone would be hollow, unless they grafted bone from my hip or put in a metal plate. They weren't sure of the course of action because they would not be able to see the extent of the damage until they had bored down through flesh to open the bone.

The night before the surgery we stayed in a hotel in Seattle near the Space Needle, built for the World's Fair my parents had attended as children. We walked out to the old fairgrounds and bought roundtrip tickets for the Monorail, played games on the midway, then walked into the old Armory building that had a food court. We rode the Bubbleator, looked at the shops, and I was allowed to eat anything I liked because I would not be able to have real food for at least a month. There was a chance I might never taste anything properly again. We had big, greasy burgers with fries and shakes, cotton candy, caramel apples. Back at the hotel I sat down with a spoon from home and licked my way through a container of store-bought chocolate frosting while my mother watched the first part of *The Thorn Birds*. At bedtime I was ill with expectation and too much food and locked myself in the bathroom, pressing my face against cool, gray tiles that smelled of antiseptic spray.

Early the next morning my father drove us to the hospital and dropped us at the front door. I was silent as the nurses prepped me for surgery. I swallowed pills to make me sleepy, tucked my hands under the crisp sheets, fell asleep shivering, and woke that evening in intensive care.

Surfacing from the drugs, I could hear a television but I could not move. My head had been pulverized and I started to panic. This was worse than any nightmare, worse than any monster under the bed. I sucked air through my nose and would have moaned or cried but literally could not. My eyes were glued together, but after a few minutes I was able to pry them open and stare out through eyelashes crusty with some kind of yellow adhesive. My mother was only thirty years old but she had streaks of gray in her shiny brown hair. She was watching the second part of *The Thorn Birds* on the television above my bed, and one of her hands gripped the rail next to my hip. Her face was turned up toward the television, watching Richard Chamberlain move in to kiss Rachel Ward.

Reaching up with tentative fingers, I found that my face was swollen into a perfectly round shape. The inside of my mouth was full of blood, and my tongue rubbed against cotton packed into the incision. Nurses came and rolled me around. My mother was there and then gone. It was night, then day, then night again, and I was alone in intensive care and my head was exploding. Someone showed up next to me and said that I must talk. I forced sound out—not words, but grunts—around my swollen tongue and cracked lips, tasting the anesthesia and blood-soaked gauze, my cheeks ripping against the metal wire clamping my teeth together.

The doctor who came to change the surgical dressing the next morning leaned forward and breathed in my face, the mingled scent of cigarettes and tomato juice making me gag as he reached in my mouth, reeling the long, blood-soaked dressing out of the deep hole. He gave me a huge syringe with a curved plastic tip and told me to plunge it in the wound each day, sending water down the hole to irrigate it.

I went back to school within a few days of leaving intensive care. I talked after a fashion, moving my lips circumspectly. I only ate what could be siphoned with a straw through clenched teeth.

It was disgusting to do, and even worse to watch. The other kids made fun of me, so I largely gave up food.

I ate perhaps half a cup of chocolate pudding each day. My grandmother made broth when I visited the farm, and I waited for the steaming fluid to cool before taking small sips. I dabbed wax on the wires to protect my cheeks and poked medication through the gap left by the teeth removed in the surgery.

Within four weeks I lost over one-third of my body weight. My arms and legs were skeletal and my face and hands turned a greenish-yellow color. My mother was frantically worried, mashing food and putting bowls of porridge in front of me. She bought nutritional supplements and protein drinks and I pushed all the offerings away. I did not want to eat. I said that I was *fine* and threatened to run away if she took me to the doctor again.

Everything seemed gray and lustrous. I slept. I dreamed. I starved.

lucky

As the hours passed I started to feel dizzy and shake. Finally I wobbled over to a nurse and said, "I'm sorry, but I'm going to pass out," and listed to the side, drooping across the counter. There were still no exam rooms available, but he found me a gurney in a quiet hallway and I curled up in the fetal position, covering my face with both hands.

Byron and the boy found chairs and sat next to me with stricken expressions, reading *The Borrowers* out loud.

Late in the afternoon a different nurse found me still parked in the hallway on a gurney and I was wheeled into an exam room. The nurse took a brief history and then asked, "On a scale of one to ten, if one means no pain and ten is the worst pain you have ever experienced, what is this pain like?"

I hate the one-to-ten scale. I especially hate the illustrated versions with smiling faces running to frowning faces. What relevance does it have? What symbolic value? Does the pain of a broken pelvis even compare to the pain of childbirth? Does an eyelid slashed open, blood gushing down your face, have any relevance to a violently bruised heart? Can you contrast grief with despair? The answer is no. The only way for me to honestly convey information on a scale would be to assign my own values, but medical staff do not want qualified or poetic answers.

"The pain I am experiencing now is almost as bad as the time I had gangrene in my stomach," I replied. Did I have gangrene? *In my stomach*? Someone said so, but who? I was too overwhelmed to put the facts together or explain. The pain in my abdomen was monstrous and hours in the hospital had moved me no closer to relief.

"I've never known her to admit to feeling bad," Byron added, and the nurse blinked and then started to hurry through her routines.

She tried to start an IV and encountered my perniciously small veins, always a problem but even more difficult when I am dehydrated and in crisis. It took several minutes of tracking old scars and thumping viscous skin to find a suitable location. She worried aloud that the needle was not big enough to do some of the tests I might need later in the day.

Moving to the other arm, she tried to take some blood, but the first attempt missed. The second worked, but she came back moments later to say that the blood had clotted before it made it to the lab. Her hands were shaking by the time the third blood draw clotted, and the fourth was performed by another technician rushed in from somewhere else in the building to help. He had to roll the vials continuously to keep the blood in whatever state was required for testing.

The lab tech asked, "Does your blood always clot like this?"

"Whatever should not happen will," I replied.

A doctor appeared and asked a few questions. I was far too sick to adequately describe my complicated history and vaguely fluttered my hand instead of giving crisp facts and data. My mouth and brain would not cooperate, could not offer up the names of my diseases. Did they have names, I wondered? No, they are just a series of disconnected nonsensical phrases and memories.

The doctor frowned when I said, "The big thing you should know is that an infection in my stomach nearly killed me—or did kill me, depending on who you ask."

The doctor looked at Byron. He nodded confirmation that the story was true. The doctor stood up and announced that I had to get an ultrasound immediately. I closed my eyes and tried to count backwards from 100.

In March of 1983, I woke up feeling ill and asked to stay home. It had been eight weeks since the cancer surgery, four weeks since the surgery on my jaw, and my mouth was still wired shut. My mother was putting on makeup in the bathroom and she felt my forehead. I didn't have a fever so she said no; I had missed too much school already.

In the middle of a lesson on the slave trade and disputed expansion of Western territories, I knew I was going to throw up and ran from the classroom.

I reached the girl's rest room just as a fluid breakfast gushed up from my stomach, filling my mouth but found no exit, held back by the boundary of wires. I was choking and strangling and then gagging and pushing the vomit up further, up and out through my nose, spraying the toilet and wall, splashing all over my clothes. Waves of nausea hit and I couldn't breathe, my esophagus and mouth and nose all full, no oxygen getting through, my breath completely gone.

Finally it stopped for a moment and I fell to the floor, sucking air through the wire mesh, through sinuses and a nose singed with stomach acids, unable to stand up or call for help or do anything but feel the cold certainty of the scratched yellow tiled floor.

If I had been granted a wish in that moment it would not have been for salvation but for death. This was simply not fair. I had cancer, I had some other weird thing wrong with the bones of my face, and now this indignity. It was too much, simply unbearable, but there was no way to escape. I vomited through my nose over and over.

Snorting and covered with filth, lying on the damp floor, I looked around the cubicle, at the shining chrome of the toilet handle and the orange metal stalls, and knew with dull conviction that children do not choke to death on their own vomit in elementary school bathrooms.

A girl named Angie found me crouched on the floor, spew erupting from my nose. She touched my back and patted my face with a damp paper towel and led me to the office.

The secretary looked up from her electric typewriter and frowned when she saw me. We had not been on good terms for many years; she was certain my perpetual bad health was a performance, even as I turned in notes from surgeons.

"She was puking through her nose!" Angie exclaimed, and I swayed and grasped the edge of the desk. The secretary recoiled and then gestured with one hand toward the yellow vinyl bench in the office, picking up the phone with the other.

As an adult, I have to wonder why the secretary did not call an ambulance; certainly, I could have died that afternoon. But because the school secretary was not overly concerned, my father dropped me off at home alone. He had to go back to work. I crawled into bed and my dog jumped in with me, his little body shaking as I vomited through my nose, only just barely finding the energy to roll over and grab the bowl each time the nausea hit. There wasn't enough oxygen getting through the miasma, and I hung my head over the bed, trying to breathe, trying not to throw up again. Eventually my body could not produce even an ounce of bile, and I dry heaved through the day, wishing myself hollow like a stacking doll.

My mother was horrified when she came home from work. I refused to eat or drink anything for fear of what might happen, and finally, after two days, I ended up in the hospital, diagnosed with malnutrition, hooked up to an intravenous supply of food.

The surgeon wanted to cut the wires on my teeth, but other specialists told him that my jaw was like glass and that the slightest disturbance was risky. The nurse who tucked me into bed, however, didn't wait to get directions from a doctor. Gasping at the image of a child alone, choking on vomit, her hands moved decisively toward the wire cutters the surgeon had put on a hook above the bed. "Hold still," she said, then pulled my dry, cracked lips open and delicately snipped each wire.

I opened my mouth for the first time in a month, the joints groaning, the mush of my inner cheeks smarting from days of sickness. I put my hands over my face and smiled.

When I was released from the hospital, jaw creaking, the doctors were certain that I would recover quickly now that I could eat solid food. They thought I had a stomach virus; they said it was not related to the cancer or the cyst. My mother set me up on the couch with the rainbow-colored afghan knitted by my great-grandmother and the television remote. She found a TV tray and made me a root beer float. Casper was on my lap and I held on to my stuffed lion. There was a dull, throbbing pain in my lower belly, but I was not about to tell anyone. I curled up on the couch, pulling my legs up around the secret.

I drifted in and out of sleep watching *Have Gun Will Travel*. My parents were talking to a salesman about vinyl siding. They sat at the round wooden kitchen table discussing pricing and color options.

The pain in my stomach was getting worse every minute but I ignored it. During a commercial break I shuffled my dog to the side, moved to get up, and felt my stomach being ripped in half by an invisible dagger. It was a transcendent feeling that was beyond anything before, beyond terror, beyond tears.

I fell back on the couch, staring up at the framed photographs on the wall, at the coat rack decoupaged with butterflies, through the window framing pine trees in the front yard. The salesman continued his pitch; my parents sat with their backs to me. Casper whimpered and pushed his face into my palm.

After five or ten minutes I got up slowly and shuffled off to my bedroom, crawled into the white-canopied bed, and went to sleep. I thought if I put the blanket over my head they wouldn't notice.

Over the next two days my mother hovered over the bed, coaxing me to eat. She sent my father out to the store for ice cream and soda, but I kept turning my head away. I just wanted to sleep. She said that I needed to go to the doctor but I said no, I was *fine*, there was no problem. She took my temperature, watched the number going up every hour, and finally pulled me out of bed and walked me to the car. I was too weak to stand up straight or navigate the pebbled path without assistance. She put me in the back of the Buick and I lay across the seat, looking at the tops of trees blurring green, the blackness of the old quarry, the small waterfalls, smelling the salty ruin of low tide. The Olympic Mountains stood majestically over the trees and water, impassively watching the humans below. My mother drove me around the inlet and across the peninsula to see a surgeon.

The doctor barely touched my hand before he understood. There was no lengthy examination. My appendix had exploded. During the forty-eight hours I refused to get out of bed, the infection had spread through my abdomen and the various systems of my body were shutting down. I was dying. He told my mother to take me straight to the hospital, straight to surgery. I said no, tried to argue, but I was too weak. I suggested going home for my things, thinking that a delay might take me closer to my goal of oblivion. He shook his head and asked the nurse to cancel his other appointments.

They dosed me with anesthesia and told me to count backwards. *Ten, nine, eight, seven, six,* my head filled with the smell of rubber and my veins flooded with cold, and then I was asleep.

I woke up to the sight of more stuffed animals and flowers lining the windowsill, to the familiar stink of ammonia and urine, latex and sweat. I was back in the children's ward, staring at the mural of the leering farm maiden and her poorly drawn red barn. Pulling the blue hospital gown away from my clammy body, I looked at the new scar, six inches long, puckered skin stapled and taped shut, greenish fluid leaking through the cracks. There were blisters the size of silver dollars erupting underneath the tape. I pulled myself up, then used my hands to push limp and unwilling legs off the bed. Grabbing the IV pole, I lurched over to a chair and let myself drop down on the cracked vinyl, the hospital gown edging up to reveal bony legs covered in bruises from the medical staff yanking me across the gurney onto the operating table.

When the nurse came to take my temperature she was surprised to find me up, but congratulated me and asked if I wanted food. She brought me foul salty broth and red Jell-O. I had a roommate with a broken leg and she wanted to watch an episode of *Little House on the Prairie*. Albert left a smoking pipe in the basement of the blind school, setting the place on fire, killing Mrs. Garvey and Mary's baby.

That night I felt something fetid spreading through my belly. I turned on my side and said I was *fine* each time the nurse came to see me. She put a clean plastic cover on a glass thermometer and took my temperature; it kept going up. My stomach started to balloon out.

The doctor came back near dawn. He pulled up the hospital gown, put his hand on my belly, and said that the infection must have spread; he said that I had to be very brave, that I needed more surgery.

The hospital was quiet and dark. I could hear my roommate whispering in her sleep. I could see car lights reflected against the mural, trailing across the farm scene, the animals with their baleful smiles.

I said *no* and he said if I didn't have surgery, I would die. But I knew that I would die no matter what, and didn't want them to cut me open again. If I had been able to walk, I would have left the hospital, but the fever kept rising—something rank was destroying my guts and I was ruinously weak.

My mother arrived just as they wheeled me out of the room. She stood next to my gurney in the special patient's elevator, larger than the ones used for visitors, with metal floors and padded walls. She held my hand and I looked up at her and began to describe the kind of funeral I wanted. Nurses and orderlies shushed me and my mother looked like she had just been punched in the face. I said *goodbye*; I meant *forever*.

The surgery took hours longer than predicted. I went under refusing to count or talk to anyone, concerned with only one thing: death. I didn't want to wake up.

In the surgical recovery room, the nurses had to scream and scream to make me angry enough to fight back, to argue, to survive.

The scar from the second stomach surgery is a foot long and two inches wide in places; my abdomen was so distended it was impossible to put me together properly. Internal organs were pulled out, scoured, and gently laid back in place. The infection and surgery left a web of scar tissue around the organs, binding them together.

The surgeon said that I was lucky. He said that someone so sick had no resources to fight a septic infection and survive two major abdominal surgeries. He said that healthy adults die from less serious complications. I stared up at him, pain and rage choking off any possible reply. My body was just a slab of clay for the nurses and doctors to move around.

Standing next to the hospital bed, he picked up my hand and leaned close. "I need to say this because I don't think anyone else will. Your mother has done everything possible for you. She thinks you are her greatest accomplishment. Please don't let her down."

During the first week in the hospital my mother washed my face with a washcloth, smoothed the lank greasy hair back from my forehead, fed me chips of ice. I could not move at all, not even to turn on my side. The IV put food and drugs in my system, and a catheter drained urine out. It took seven days to figure out how to make my legs cooperate enough to bend my knees.

Eventually the nurses heaved me up, wrapped my torso in plastic, and put me in the shower. I held on to a metal bar, stooped over, eyes closed, the water running down my back and sputtering against the plastic shield. My mother wanted to help but I said no, shut the door; after the shower I dried myself with a towel, patting the bits of my body within reach, feeling like nothing was connected any longer. It took half an hour to dry off, put on a fresh gown, and shuffle back to bed.

The new incisions split open, bursting with blisters and pus. I developed an allergy to the adhesive holding pieces of my body together, to the sheets on the bed, to the pain medication intended to help me rest. The intravenous line had to be moved constantly from arm to arm, hand to hand, as each site swelled with infection. Days and nights passed in a feverish, drug-induced torpor. Eventually I refused to take pain medication, no matter how much the nurses frowned and coaxed, and if they tried to inject something in my IV, I threatened to pull the line out.

My teacher brought the whole class to visit and they clustered around, staring down at me with curious faces. The other kid with a remarkable disease, something that made his tongue pulpy and distorted, explored the room and then crawled behind the bed and into the springs. The teacher gave me C.S. Lewis books about space travel to read during my convalescence.

When I left the hospital one month later it was April and I was still just twelve years old, a sixth grader, not too old to play with dolls. I had a little white dog, dutiful parents, a nice teacher and a friend named Angie. I had a scar bisecting the front of my neck, a hole in my jaw, and a swollen mess of a belly.

We stopped at the store and my mother picked out new clothes that would not chafe against my healing incisions. At home I opened the scrapbook decorated with a picture of the wobbly headed creature from the film *E.T.* and pasted the new hospital bracelet next to all the others.

spoiled

Byron and the boy were still reading about the adventures of the miniature people in *The Borrowers* when the emergency room doctor came back with a benediction: At four in the afternoon I was finally injected with anti-nausea medication. The particular brand they chose did not diminish my convulsive dry heaves, but it did make me sleepy just in time to go to ultrasound.

It is never clear when the person pushing your gurney from one place to the next will want to talk; I was not feeling well enough to chat so I closed my eyes during the transport from the ER to the radiology department. When I arrived, the technician asked me to roll on my back and then pressed a wand against my swollen organs. The medication let sleep intervene, and I drifted into a familiar medical routine, letting the staff push me around like putty as I half-listened to their directions and played records in my mind. The technician asked all sorts of questions that I did not want to answer: Have you ever had stomach infections? *Yes*. Surgery? *Yes*. Complications? *Yes*. Why? Silence. Has anyone ever mentioned that there is something unusual about your digestive system? *Yes, and I'm tired of that story.*

Somewhere in my murky sleep I realized that the test was taking too long, that she kept asking me to shift for new views of the same area. She was recording trouble spots, circling things on the screen. I wondered if she had found cancer, wondered if I would survive this hospitalization.

I woke up finally and shuddered at the sticky, cold fluid the technician smoothed across the squishy, distorted plane of my stomach. The pain was simply intolerable, but after that first sober shiver I pulled back my shoulders and set my teeth. Long before I was diagnosed with cancer I learned to hold my breath long enough to get a perfect full-body scan. I learned to hold still as instruments were pressed on my eyes, as needles shot electricity through my muscles and nerves, as pieces of skin were burned with chemicals.

It was not fair to be short with the lab technician examining my body. It wasn't her fault that the tests reminded me of the past. I turned on my side so she could find a better view of the suspect organs.

Back downstairs in the ER, Byron tried to distract me from what was happening. He reported that the woman in the examination room next to mine had an argument with an armed security guard, screaming that she was a police officer and would "kick his ass."

When I didn't laugh, he stroked my hair and asked, "Do you want me to call your mother?"

LESSONS IN TAXIDERMY   53

I flinched. "No, please don't. It will upset her. If she calls the house for some reason, don't even tell her."

"Are you sure?"

"She has been through too much. I don't want her to worry."

Our son looked tired and I asked if he wanted to go home. He nodded, patted my hand, and I leaned forward to kiss his cheek. I thanked him for staying with me and he smiled with a shy and contemplative expression. Most kids would have been upset or disruptive. His sister would have told lengthy comic monologues, charming the staff. At age seven this little boy had the natural gravity of an elderly gentleman from another era. He would have been more scared not to know what was happening, but a day patiently sitting by my side was more than enough.

Byron said, "I'll find someone to take the kids. I'll be back later."

"You can stay home with them, I'm OK here alone," I replied.

He shook his head at me and said, "I'll be back. Promise that you will tell them the truth?"

I nodded and waved as they walked away down the corridor.

The doctor came back with the radiology report: The blood tests and ultrasound offered conflicting information. "It looks like you might need surgery," he said.

One of the military laboratories on the East Coast determined that my cancer was not the variety local doctors had supposed. The surgeon said that the cause of the disease was still a mystery, that the specific type of cancer was unheard of in a child, but that I should not worry; he had removed all of the

diseased tissue. The diagnosis was downgraded from terminal
to malignant.

I had missed most of the end of elementary school without
doing any of the assigned work, but my teacher shrugged; he
asked me to tutor younger children who did not know how to
read. I spent the days drifting with the lassitude of extreme
illness, sitting on the classroom beanbag chair reading novels.
The other students in my grade were required to complete stan-
dardized competence evaluations, while I built a sundial from a
piece of plywood and a dowel and sat on the tarmac of the playground next to the tetherball posts, marking the time with a black
felt-tip pen.

When I was named valedictorian of the class, other children
muttered that I was spoiled, that I did not deserve the distinction.
The honor had nothing to do with my scholastic achievements; a
child who had not been present for the larger portion of the previous two years was obviously not the most academically rigorous
person in the class. The teachers who made the decision were
voting for me out of pity, sympathy, and true kindness. But I
would have rather earned the title.

My parents drove me off the peninsula to choose a dress for
the occasion and I stared up at the 500-foot towers of the
Narrows Bridge swooping across the sky. We went to the B&I
variety store in Tacoma and walked through the musty narrow
hallways, past the chickens who played checkers for the price of a
quarter. I stopped briefly in the pet store to admire the stacked
cages of rats, mice, guinea pigs, ferrets, snakes, cats, and dogs.
When I was younger there had been a giant cage with metal bars
housing Ivan the gorilla, who glowered down at the spectators,
pounded the walls, or sometimes sat slumped over, eyes dull, not

looking at the crowd. When the store bought him, he lived with his keeper and was brought up as if he were a human child, with smart suits and other kids to play with. He rode in cars and performed at public events. But when he grew too large he was moved to a cage with bars, and there he sat for thirty years.

None of the dresses I tried on fit properly. My body was still raw and misshapen from surgery, arms and legs bony from malnutrition. One dress after another was pulled over my head, but they all looked fundamentally wrong on me. They were too long, or too short, or a color that contrasted badly with my blue-green skin tone. Some were cut straight up and down, which didn't work with my bulging stomach. Others were voluminous poufs, which emphasized the awkwardness of my body. I was just trying to cover my scars, and it seemed cruel that I could not find a dress that fit.

Finally, buried deep on a sales rack, there was a dress that had probably sat unwanted and neglected in the store for years. It was white, decorated with a rainbow print, and draped like my grandmother's square-dancing dresses: tight at the waist but flaring out, with plenty of material to cover my gaunt legs and emaciated arms. The garment fit perfectly, and it was pretty clear nobody else would have the same dress.

After we paid we went to the arcade, which had video games and air hockey tables and a water slide. I rode the old carousel, spinning around and around, the view of a busy Tacoma road blurring through the windows. Next we stopped in the toy section and my mother said that I could pick out anything I wanted; if it was too expensive, she would put the item on layaway.

The kids at school were correct in saying that I was spoiled. My parents worked overtime every single day, typing and filing, pumping gas and cleaning toilets, to pay my medical bills.

Whatever was left was devoted to amusing me. I was allowed to have any material possession my family could afford to buy. I was taken on trips. I never had to do chores or eat my grandmother's rice pudding. I even grew to believe that I was entitled to these privileges. But nobody made any effort to disguise the motivation behind the acts of charity. I was coddled because I was sick, spoiled because I was rotting from the inside out.

During the elementary school graduation ceremony I announced the various performances and awards. The class sang the Neil Diamond song "America," "The Rainbow Connection" from *The Muppet Movie*, and "Climb Ev'ry Mountain" from *The Sound of Music*. My voice was frayed, ruined from the surgery on my neck, so I mouthed the words as the other children sang. I wanted to believe the injunction of Mother Superior, wanted to follow every byway until I found my dream.

Sitting with the other children on the orange carpeting of the auditorium, waiting for our names to be called to receive graduation certificates, my hands strayed to my neck. I prodded each side, meticulously avoiding the scar. There was not supposed to be a problem. But my fingers found a lump and, sitting there waiting for my name to be called, I knew that I was touching cancer.

Nobody except my mother believed me; that summer she took me to the doctors over and over again and they all poked my neck and shook their heads. They said that there was no chance the cancer had spread. Some of the doctors were eyeing my mother suspiciously, speaking to her in a way that conveyed disdain. They seemed to think we were making up stories.

I kept insisting that something was wrong, and my reward was to sit shivering in the corridors of hospitals, telling each person I met that I knew the cancer had spread. Finally one surgeon listened and agreed to do a biopsy. He was making a concession that might upset the insurance company; he said that even if the cancer had come back, it would be minor.

I went to have my teeth cleaned and X-rays showed that there were more cysts in my jaw. The doctors needed to operate fast to prevent more devastation in the bone. During that surgery my mouth was slowly wrenched open, instruments holding it beyond the stress point. The cartilage of the joints started to slip.

One week later I had surgery to remove the lump in my neck. I could not open my mouth wide enough to allow the anesthesiologist to establish a breathing tube. While I was under sedation the jaw was cracked open, destroying what was left of the cartilage.

The surgeon said that when he opened my neck the lymph nodes were gray and sodden with disease, visibly malignant, that I should have had the surgery months earlier. He said that the disease had been allowed to progress too long, that I would now have to be subjected to even more rigorous tests and treatments. He said that the cancer might spread throughout my body.

After the first year of surgeries my parents took me on a trip to California. We drove down the coast, past the ocean beaches, through the redwood forests. We went to Knott's Berry Farm, Great America, and Disneyland. We went to the Winchester Mystery House, a mansion built with the fortune earned from the repeating rifle. The widow of the inventor used up decades and immense sums of money to create a fantastic, elaborate dwelling with secret passages and false staircases. She thought that if she kept building, the ghosts of the people killed by the guns would not be able to find her.

During a follow-up appointment with the oral surgeon, I settled in the beige reclining examination chair and asked, "How can it possibly be true that none of these diseases are related to each other?"

He shook his head in exasperation; he wanted to give me an answer. He turned on the light to look at the new X-ray of my jaw, then paused. "Do you have any moles?" he asked.

I blinked at him and replied, "A couple, but mostly I just have skin tags."

He banged his hand on the counter and looked at my mother. "Skin tags? Why didn't you tell me?"

She narrowed her eyes at him. "Why didn't you *ask*? She's been seeing a dermatologist for ten years. It's all in her charts."

He spun in his chair and rolled over to where I was sitting. "Show me," he demanded, and I pulled down the collar of my shirt.

The oral surgeon was silent as he stared at the front of my neck, then asked me to turn and show my back.

I had been under the care of a dermatologist since age three. He thought the skin tags were fascinating, extraordinary, because no matter how often he treated me they always came back. At first I had to be dosed with tranquilizers before the appointments, but by age seven I didn't need the drugs. The dermatologist used chemicals to singe bits of skin off my body every month; although there were many hundreds of lesions on a person so young, the medical textbooks denied that they could be a serious problem. There were no documented cases of anyone that young with the problem the doctor was looking at, so he didn't see it.

Over the years I had also been treated by an endocrinologist, a neurologist, two surgeons, and a half dozen other doctors who lived on the peninsula. Specialists at five hospitals in Seattle had reviewed my case. They had all looked at my skin, all agreed that the odd lumpy things covering my torso were nothing to worry about. The white and clear and red bumps trailed across my body. They tore against the collars of my shirts or caught in the links of necklaces, bleeding and healing and growing bigger every day.

The oral surgeon pulled out a pen to start making notes. "That is cancer," he said to my mother. "She has skin cancer. This explains the cysts, at least. She has Gorlin's Syndrome." He pulled a heavy medical dictionary down from a shelf, checked the index, and opened the book to a page with a photograph of a man's face, covered in spots that were identical to those on my back and chest.

I looked down at the book, then at my mother. She was staring at the doctor, lips pressed together, hands gripping the arms of a chair as though she wanted to jump up and run away. The room was warm but I felt like I had been rolling in a bank of snow without a coat. The doctor kept talking but I could not take it in, the list was too long, the potential side-effects too frightening.

Then he said, "But this isn't related to the other cancer."

"*How is that possible?*" I whispered.

"I don't know."

Within a week, a new dermatologist had been located to deal with the skin cancer. He stood on a stool and wore a magnifying glass on his head like a coal miner's lantern. He scrutinized every inch of my torso, excited to have a case for the textbooks under his control. He said there were only five other people like me on the West Coast.

It took four years of appointments to remove the tumors, a few dozen at a time; a shot for each one and then a digging, cutting motion, followed by an electrical charge to cauterize the tissue. The first dozen cuts hurt, but I learned not to feel them, not to notice, even if the doctor forgot to give me the anesthetic. I laid on scratchy white paper covering a black vinyl exam table, half-naked, staring at the ceiling and reciting the names of all the states in alphabetical order, seeing each name printed in my mind, teaching myself how to think in words instead of images. After the first hundred tumors were removed, the doctor said I was mutilated, not fit to be seen by other children. He gave me a permanent waiver to be excused from physical education at school.

There were new rules: I was not allowed to go in the sun at all. I was not allowed to swim in chlorinated water ever again. I had to keep the new scars completely dry until the scabs fell off. I was thirteen years old and not allowed to bathe. My mother washed my hair in the sink, draping towels across crusty, raw wounds. Even with my hair shiny and clean I felt dirty, unkempt, disheveled, wrong.

Whenever possible I went to school, but surgeries, appointments, and illnesses intervened. My immune system started to fail after so many years of trauma; between the ages of twelve and fourteen I had bronchitis and pneumonia on at least twenty occasions. Each time my lungs were congested, I had to have an X-ray to determine if the cancer had spread. Incapacitating headaches led to multiple CT scans because the doctors thought it likely I had brain cancer. Routine blood tests checked for leukemia and demonstrated that I had acute anemia amidst other abstruse disorders.

One day I looked down and saw that my already pale body was blanching; one of the doctors shook his head and said my immune system was destroying the pigment. My blood, though not yet streaming with cancer, had turned against me, and my heart decided that circulating hemoglobin to all extremities was no longer a priority. My hands were so cold I thought my fingers might snap off.

If anyone saw my scars, they recoiled—"What happened to you? Are those cigarette burns?" Some people assumed that I had done the damage to my own body; when I retorted with the word *cancer* they screwed up their faces and turned away in fear or disgust.

The illness was visible, incontrovertible, undeniable, and real. I suffered daily indignities for being the sick kid, the weird kid, the outcast. I would not have dared to eat in the lunchroom or congregate at the back of the school during breaks. Random luck had given me the art teacher for homeroom and she didn't mind if I stayed in the supply closet reading a comic strip called *Life in Hell*.

There were moments of sanity, some tenuous connections to other people. I made friends with a girl in art class; her name was Elizabeth and we used the school facilities to produce an underground newspaper. Amy sat next to me in typing class and offered to share candy when the teacher wasn't looking. In homeroom there was a boy named Teddy with tasseled loafers and Izod shirts; we sat on high stools, giggling during the Pledge of Allegiance. Angie went to a different school but sometimes she came to visit, or I would get a ride to watch her playing the flute in marching band. But as the months passed and the illness worsened, even those people I considered friends faded in my mind, turning into ghosts.

I wanted to be invisible, and figured out that if I did not respond, most people would leave me alone. A boy named David sat in front of me in a couple of classes and he made it a daily habit to taunt and tease. The girls in the seats around me laughed at whatever he said, but I could not even hear the words. I just looked straight into his eyes, never blinking, never changing my blank expression. After a few months he faltered, and his face flushed red like a crayon. He looked down, turned away.

No matter what happened I looked straight ahead and the people around me receded. I walked alone through an amorphous blur of hallways, imagining the other kids swirling down a drain like dirty bath water.

The adults in charge of the junior high school believed I was malingering. I had to do twice as much work to compensate for absences, and even then was not able to keep up because teachers subtracted points off my total grade for every missed day. The guidance counselor read my physical education waiver and told me that I was a hypochondriac. The math teacher would not accept late work under any circumstance. One day the English teacher refused to accept my note for an absence. "If you want to succeed in life, you have to show up," she said. The whole class was watching as she continued, "This is simply unacceptable. Why do you think you can get away with this?"

I did not know what to say. I whispered, "*I have cancer.*"

She tossed the note on to her desk and crossed her arms. "Prove it," she hissed.

I was wearing a white turtleneck and red sweatshirt. Without pausing to think, I yanked both up, past my shoulders, showing her the proof she required. Her face went pale as she looked at the long, deep gashes visible above the waist of my jeans, at the hundreds of surgical welts marring my torso. The other kids could see the scars on my back. The room was absolutely silent as the teacher leaned forward and signed the note.

The doctors kept sending me from one hospital to the next in pursuit of ever more esoteric potions and cures. During the tests

I could spend hours each day tracing shapes with the eye that moved, leaving the other fixed on a point in the distance, watching objects dance and blur.

After one procedure the doctor wanted to keep me in the hospital for a week; he said that my bodily fluids would be radioactive. I pleaded with him to let me go home. He agreed but said that I had to use plastic cutlery and paper plates, and flush three times after using the toilet. But even after issuing these ominous guidelines, he insisted that the tests were not dangerous and would cause no side effects.

Within a few weeks, my hair started to fall out. I woke up each day to a pillow covered with hair; when I brushed it in the morning, huge chunks came away in my hand.

During an appointment at the children's hospital in the city, a doctor finally realized that I only knew the answer to the question "How many fingers am I holding up?" by dividing the number viewed by a factor of two. He said I needed surgery. I said no, refused, but they promised that I could go home directly afterward, that it would be minor, that it wouldn't hurt very much. They scheduled the appointment during spring vacation so I wouldn't miss any school, and as my parents drove me to the city I sat in the backseat listening to *Purple Rain* on my Walkman.

The doctors did not explain the unique pain achieved by having your eyeball popped out of its socket, moved to the side, and a major muscle spliced. Waking up in recovery, it felt like they had driven a sledgehammer through my eye socket. I was hustled out of bed by a nurse, then shuffled out to my parents' car clutching a wet towel to my face. The overcast day was a shattering, surging burst of color ripping my mind apart.

Back at home I looked in the mirror and saw that my eye was bloodied and bruised all the way to the iris. When would this vanish? My mother called the hospital; they said it might take six months. I replied that I was not going back to school, ever, and she looked at my eye and sighed. "You are too young to drop out. It's illegal."

"I don't care. I'm never going back again."

For the first time I could see everything directly, and this left me bereft and angry. It was exponentially harder to read, write, or even walk. The plane of the world had shifted; I had no depth perception, to the degree that I could not open a cupboard door without hitting my face with the knob. I had learned to ride a bicycle with double vision, but could not summon enough balance to ride with normal vision.

One evening I watched a made-for-television movie called *Surviving: A Family in Crisis*. The plot featured Molly Ringwald playing a disturbed girl with a death fixation and I watched carefully as she schemed to end her life. This seemed like an excellent idea, but our garage was too drafty to set up an asphyxiation. The stove was electric, not gas. Hanging was out of the question: All my books about frontier justice made it clear that the method was not efficient. The only drugs in the house were antibiotics and I was already allergic to them—the most I could get out of an overdose was a really bad rash. I considered fire; there were accelerants in the garage, but what if I just ended up in the hospital with a terrible burn? That would be pointless. Biology lessons and countless blood draws had taught me that arteries are buried too deep to reach without a really good tool; there were no sharp knives in the house, and I didn't live within walking distance of a store. I couldn't think of any method that would definitely end in death, and didn't want to go to the hospital after a botched attempt, with adults looming over me assuming my actions were a cry for help.

I didn't want help. If I needed to express an emotion, it was a pure and refined rage. One day I locked myself in the bathroom with a pair of scissors and my father's rusty, disposable safety razor. I chopped what was left of my hair short and then slowly dragged the razor across my scalp, skin and blood coming away with the hair.

On the morning I should have gone back to school I sat with my back against my bedroom door, rubbing my stubbly crusty scalp, refusing to come out. My parents stood on the other side knocking, but I ignored them. Later in the week, after it became clear that my strike against school could not be addressed with threats and bribes, my mother took me to see the nice lady doctor who looked after my endocrine system.

I sat on the exam table, feeling the paper cover shift as I pulled my feet up to sit cross-legged. The doctor was wearing a skirt and Birkenstock sandals under her lab coat. She waved a flashlight in front of my eyes, felt my neck, listened as my mother described the odd behavior of her recalcitrant child. The doctor patted my hand and asked, "What are we going to do with you?"

"I'm not going back to school. I don't care what you say. If you make me, I'll burn the place down."

She shook her head and started to make notes in my chart. "Maybe you should have a small rest. I can sign you out of school but you have to promise me something."

This was a surprise; she could actually take me out of school? I wished that I had known years earlier. I nodded.

"First of all, you will have to go to counseling every week. Secondly, I want you to promise that you won't scare your mother anymore. OK?"

I shrugged. That seemed fair enough. The doctor left the room to write a letter to the superintendent of schools, placing me in a state-funded homeschooling program. Later that week, my father dropped me off for the first appointment with a therapist. For the next six months I sat in her office once a week for fifty-minute sessions. She stared at me, and I stared at an ornamental ceramic elephant in the corner of the room. We never had a single conversation. When the insurance ran out, my mother asked me what therapy was like and I described the process. She asked if it was worth sixty-five dollars to sit silently staring at decorative pottery and I reckoned it wasn't. I did not go back for another appointment.

Most days I slept for twenty hours, waking only long enough to eat a can of ravioli. The school district sent a tutor to my house every Thursday afternoon and I would drag myself out of bed to let him in, never bothering to change out of pajamas. It was the same man who had been the playground monitor at my elementary school and he would place his leather gloves on the wooden kitchen chair, then sit down on top of them. He never took off his winter coat, no matter what the season. It took about an hour to correct the previous week's work and set the assignments for the next. I always offered him a Diet Coke and listened to his comments, and after he left I locked the door and went back to bed.

The doctor had only asked me to show up for therapy and

stop scaring my mother; these were easy promises and I would keep them. But I was too tired to do more than what had been stipulated.

The homework assigned each week was completed by my mother.

maternal impression

An hour after I was moved upstairs to a ward for preoperative patients, the knot in my stomach dissolved. For the first time in twenty hours I could lie down and take a deep breath. I debated getting dressed and walking out but could not find my shoes.

A surgical resident showed up next to the bed. He was young and had trendy, horn-rimmed glasses and wore a T-shirt under his white lab coat.

He paged through the chart and then asked me to tell him about my life over the last few months, about my daily routine.

"I've been fairly decadent, I suppose, traveling around and staying out late and eating poorly." Not something to hide if surgery is imminent. Too late now to claim that I take vitamins, exercise, and enjoy sound sleep.

The doctor squinted at my dress, cat's-eye spectacles, ratty multicolored hair, the smudged black eyeliner I had not managed to clean off the night before. "What were you doing immediately before the symptoms started?"

"I was at an art show."

He turned his head to the side, fixing his eyes on the curtain around the bed, and said, "I need to ask about your drug history. Have you ever used heroin?"

"No."

"Cocaine?"

"No."

"Marijuana?"

"No."

He looked skeptical.

"Truly, the only drugs I encounter come to me through a prescription or an IV." I waved my hand for emphasis. "But I never take those if I can avoid it." If I had felt better I would have told him a charming anecdote about how nobody has even *offered* me drugs. He still looked doubtful and I shrugged. "It's true."

Years of my childhood had been spent drifting in a haze derived from big brown bottles of codeine cough syrup, tranquilizers, sedatives, fat white pain pills, shots of morphine flooding my veins. The drugs were prescribed and necessary, but at a young age I recognized that drugs were seductive, changing my perception of the world, dulling not just the pain but every physical sensation. I felt my brain striate, marbelize, bend, and swoon as my body required ever higher doses of drugs to achieve even minimal relief. The drugs made it hard to tell the difference between dreams and reality, made it impossible to concentrate and learn and remember. I was twelve years old when I stopped taking drugs and to this day, although I never discuss the issue, people do not reveal their habits or addictions in my presence.

I was calm enough to give a precise account of my medical history. By the time he weeded through the genetic disorder, cancers, auto-immune disease, pathological gastrointestinal complications, and perilous pregnancies, he was expressing concern about keeping me on the surgery schedule. He wondered if it would be possible to get my original charts; he wondered if the diagnosis might be wrong.

"Why would you have bleeding ulcers at age nine?" he asked. "What caused your chronic kidney infections?" He exclaimed over the antibiotic-resistant strep infection that lasted for ten years, increasingly bewildered by each fact I could dredge up out of the murky past. With each new revelation, he repeated, "But why?" with a thoughtful frown. Then he uttered the oft-repeated and meaningless refrain, "But that is *unheard of*."

When he finished filling two sheets of paper with notes, he found it hard to mask his excitement. He smiled and said, "You have a *fascinating* history!"

I closed my eyes after he left the room, not wanting to remember the details of what had happened, or sift through all the random scraps of information to put together a complete picture for a new set of doctors. Talking about the memories just made me tired and sad.

Nurses and technicians came to the room every forty-five minutes to take blood or vital signs, interrupting whatever bits of sleep I could grab. Somewhere in the middle of the night a room-mate appeared and she gasped *pain, pain, pain* every few minutes.

Eventually they gave her narcotics and I drifted to sleep listening to her breathe rhythmically under the sway of drugs.

Whenever my body confounded the doctors on the peninsula my parents had to take time off work. They drove me out of the woods, over the bridges I knew by the names my grandparents used—Old and New—and through a town neatly divided by an inlet I had never heard referred to by name at all. We drove past the public housing projects we lived in when I was little, parked in a dirt lot, and walked down to the old, rickety ferry terminal. The state ferry docked next to the big cranes and cavernous buildings of a naval installation where secret things happened with ships and chemicals.

One of my routine appointments was at the nuclear medicine department in a public hospital on Beacon Hill in Seattle. During each appointment the director of the lab had a cigar clenched between his teeth.

"At some point the strands of your DNA just missed a connection," he said around the cigar, and demonstrated by holding two hairy fists together with three fingers touching, the fourth set of knuckles out of order. But he couldn't explain why it happened and he couldn't tell me how a dominant genetic disorder could show up with no prior history in the family.

"You're a first generation mutation," he said. "We don't know how much radiation to give you and we are going to estimate on the high side. You probably won't be able to have children. But even if you can, you shouldn't. It would be wrong."

There is no proof of what happened to my DNA, no easy way to account for it. The peninsula plays host to six military installations. In my grandparents' generation, ships used for atom bomb testing at Bikini Atoll were brought to the naval shipyard and sandblasted, the workers wearing simple overalls and no protective gear. Nuclear waste was dumped directly into the bay, and therefore circulated throughout the Puget Sound and all the inland waterways of my hometown. Some of the ships were never completely cleaned before they were put back in active service. My parents and their sisters and brothers and cousins swam in those waters.

Extensive scientific research has documented the risk of exposure to ionizing radiation, and many journalists have reported on the phenomenon of cancer clusters. Government agencies always make counterclaims or simply deny the clusters exist, but no matter how many times I move, doctors representing the Department of Defense Centralized Tumor Registry track me down. They send letters and questionnaires asking for the details of my case. Twenty years after the diagnosis, I still receive unsolicited mail from doctors who have read about my genetic disorder. They ask if I will participate in their studies, help their research; would I please consider letting them have another piece of my body to study?

My own doctors did not know why I was sick. The specialists in the city suggested treatments, but could not diagnose the root cause. They were not willing to guess at a proper scientific reason for the wreckage of my genetic code, but they were more than happy to continue the appointments: They hinted through their treatment that I was an old-fashioned freak of fine interest.

As a child I sat in the library reading books that told me people once believed that misshapen babies were judgments from a deity. After the Dark Ages, however, *maternal impression* became the scientific explanation for people born with odd traits. The theory explains things simply: A mother scared by a wild rabbit would have a child with a harelip; a woman who saw animals shaking as they were slaughtered would have a child with epilepsy; women who craved strawberries would have children with strawberry birthmarks. Tom Thumb and other freaks were not allowed to perform in some European countries because government officials believed that a pregnant woman viewing a human oddity might be so traumatized that her unborn child would be marked forever.

During her pregnancy, my mother saw warships sitting in dry dock on a daily basis. She lived a half mile from the undersea naval warfare station, where nuclear warheads are assembled for submarines. When she was younger, the missiles would occasionally go missing, and the base offered a cash reward to anyone returning the shell.

Without enough facts and data to make a connection between toxic waste and cancer, I decided as a child to believe that it was the sight of the warships in the bay that caused the damage. Or perhaps it was more subtle, a combination of metaphoric factors, not just the weapons of mass destruction. Maybe my life could only be explained through the theory of maternal impression.

The best and most important element of medical trips to Seattle was on the waterfront, at a dark and crowded store selling souvenirs. Lined up around the back of the store were displays of native artifacts like totem poles and old canoes and beadwork. Glass cases held flea circuses and pins with poems written on the head alongside pictures of odd and wonderful things. There were bottles of deformed farm animals—like pigs with extra legs or heads—and two human mummies.

Another little store close to the Space Needle had even more freak show artifacts, with pictures and histories of Siamese twins, men who bicycled with no legs, and women with beards. I went to visit both of these stores every time I could convince an adult to take me, which was almost guaranteed when we went to Seattle—the treat promised for good behavior during tests and appointments.

I was fascinated by the displays, and started to collect more information from the *Guinness World Records*, *Ripley's Believe It or Not*, and *The Book of Lists*. The stories of spontaneous human combustion and children who vomited frogs from hell were intriguing, but I was most interested in the freaks.

Some of the people had disorders I knew about, but others were mysterious to me in the same way my disease was to my doctors. I was comforted by the fact that other people had been born with spectacular, unknowable damage, and that they had survived, even prospered. They didn't hide their bodies; they made people pay to look at them.

In my books, the freaks posed in pictures to demonstrate their signature traits, and looking at the old images made me think about how I was often examined by groups of doctors instead of one doctor in private. I thought about how I was made to walk naked down carpeted hallways while medical staff evaluated the way my spine moved, or the pattern of my walk, loudly discussing possible explanations for bizarre symptoms.

The first time I had full-body radioactive isotope scans in the cold public hospital on Beacon Hill, the radiology technician on duty twirled his curly brown hair and pushed his glasses up over and over, humming. He was so excited by the novel workings of my digestive system that he made two sets of prints and kept one for his private collection.

During these tests I was in glassy anguish, entering puberty with cancer in my endocrine system, malnourished from test-related fasting and surgeries and depression, radioactive isotopes flowing through my body. I wanted to sleep, but had to hold still without moving for two, three, four hours at a time, strapped to a table as the machine moved slowly back and forth over my body and the gamma-camera collected images.

If I twitched or moved, the test would have to start over again. I looked out the window at naked tree branches and played albums in my head: Blondie, the B-52's, the Clash, the Violent Femmes. Sometimes a repetitive and maudlin Muzak version of a popular song would intrude from the hospital corridors, corrupting my internal soundtrack.

After the appointments in Seattle, we took the ferry home. I often settled with a coat over my cold body, then, hands covering my face, dreamed of circuses and carnivals, places where my mutilation was a gift to display for an audience. The spotlight came up and I posed with all of the scars on my back exposed, then turned and threw my head back to show the fresh cuts across my neck.

The audience included doctors, but they had to stay in the crowd, had to pay to see my flesh. I was the one who decided what and how to show off, and the crowd murmured with excitement. A gamma-camera slide show flashed on a giant screen behind me, showing the distribution of the cancer and all the strange inner workings of my body. The audience whistled and cheered to see my spectacular damage.

road trip

A surgeon showed up at the foot of my bed around seven in the morning, waking me from an uneasy sleep. I reached for my glasses on the bedside table and pushed the button to raise the bed to a sitting position.

The doctor said that the ultrasound report was not conclusive, but it showed a swollen bile duct. He said that the problem might be gallstones, but this was not a diagnosis; with my history there could be many other causes of the symptoms. The smartest choice would be to keep me on the roster for surgery later that day.

He explained that normally the procedure is routine and performed as laparoscopy, with a video camera and small surgical instruments inserted through a series of tiny incisions. In an otherwise healthy person it would take no longer than forty-five minutes and require minimal recovery time. The severity of my internal scars, however, might cause serious complications, might mean that I was ineligible for laparoscopy. He said that even if they had to crack me open, separating large tracts of skin and muscle for extensive exploratory surgery, he still wanted me on the schedule.

The surgeon seemed nice. He was calm and kind and answered my questions. But the operation was not presented as an option; it was described as mandatory and urgent. He departed and a female surgical resident took over the conversation. She said that it is most desirable to do the surgery between attacks and gave me a rundown of the truly nasty potential complications of not going through with the procedure.

I wasn't even sure what function the gallbladder performed. Does it store bile? *Gall* carries connotations of exasperation, irritation, vexation. Is a gallbladder literally a pocket where the body harbors rancor?

I asked, "What if I wait a few days?"

"From what we can tell of the symptoms, whatever is going on is not chronic and manageable. This is an acute condition that will surely take you down again." There was also the unstated possibility that they might find something terrible when they opened me up.

The resident reviewed the notes compiled during earlier discussions and showed me the crabbed, tiny writing that her colleague had resorted to in order to make the information fit in the allocated space. She asked, "Is this a comprehensive overview?" and read out the highlights of what I had already detailed.

I wanted to laugh. Comprehensive? No. Not even cursory. If the doctors didn't have the old charts, how could they know what complications to worry about, what drugs to avoid? I'm not even

sure of my own blood type, can never keep track of the facts relevant to my wrecked body. I listened and nodded as she recited the
major diagnoses, then realized that she had not heard about the
worst thing that ever happened to me.

"No," I said. "There is more."

The doctor pursed her lips and shook her head slowly as I
gave her a brief account.

By my sixteenth birthday I had over three hundred scars on my
body. I had learned to divorce intellect from sensation, to think
instead of feel. There was no reward in my corporeal reality.
Each of my physical senses had failed me in some profound way;
every single system of my body harbored either a disease or
traces of earlier treatments, but I no longer noticed except
during medical appointments.

I went back to school again, enrolling at an enormous comprehensive high school that pulled kids from throughout the
south end of the peninsula. My genetic disorder had been diagnosed and brought to a state of détente, the cancer was under
control, and my vision had stabilized. Only the few students
who had gone to the same elementary school knew the truth, but
even if they remembered that I had been sick, they never understood the extent of the illness. They just thought I had been
absent for a while.

People were coming back into focus; the dreamy fantasies of
the illness abated and I looked around and noticed that I was not
the only person who spent an unnaturally large amount of time in
the art room. There were other people at the school who walked

home, even if it took hours, rather than ride the bus. While most kids wore heavy metal T-shirts and Levi's and permed their hair, there was another group of people who dressed in thrift-store clothes or basic black or some kind of distorted rural interpretation of the preppie style they saw in magazines. They didn't listen to mainstream music or hard rock, instead tuning their radios to the far left of the AM dial to pick up a tinny underground channel from Seattle called KJET. They stayed up late on the weekends to catch *Bombshelter Videos*, with a jumble of genres somehow corralled together under the word *alternative*.

Some of the kids were kitted out in the full Mod costume. They watched *Quadrophenia* obsessively and worked part-time pizza jobs to save up money for Vespas. Others had big, spiked mohawks, the bald portions of their stubbly scalps looking exposed and fragile. Lots of people were in bands. Some just wore flannel shirts and took a lot of drugs. The hallway at school where they all hung out at break was called the Waver Wall and I never grasped how that title had stuck; it was a ragtag assortment of goths, punks, skaters, addicts, thespians, depressives, and queer kids. There were probably only thirty of them standing or sitting in that hallway, but they had formed an autonomous subculture without having anything in common other than mutual disaffection.

It occurred to me that I could follow the example of this band of misfits. I already looked like a wraith; adding some dark eye makeup just distracted attention from my legitimate pallor. My hair was cut in an unfashionable chin-length bob, not because I liked the style but because it had only grown back that far; my scalp would still be bristly with new hair for a few more years. I still picked odd clothes to stay warm and cover the scars; it was not a big leap to let myself emphasize differences. My mother pleaded with me to buy nice things, but instead I put on layers of thermal underwear and leggings with skirts on top. I wore turtlenecks and bulky old cardigans, army surplus coats, and boots with sharp pointy metal tips. If people looked at my clothes they weren't looking at me; it was a costume, a trick, a game.

My parents bought me a car. It was older than me, with peeling paint and bullet holes in the trunk. It did not have a reverse gear and I had to carry cases of brake fluid and oil to keep it running, but now I could drive myself to school and doctors' appointments. I never felt that I was truly part of any group, even the one that had no entry requirements, but the car gave me a job, a task, a place in life: I could give my new friends rides to school.

The leftover anxiety of chronic illness translated to excessive caution on the roads, and other kids made fun of my high regard for safety. They had no idea why I drove so slowly, locked all the doors, made everyone wear seat belts. If anyone mocked me for the rules, I said, "You can walk if you don't like it."

Angie, Elizabeth, Teddy, Amy, and a few other people who had always been kind to me also gravitated toward the hallway. We threw parties, went to Seattle for concerts, rode ferries out to distant islands, or hung out in parking lots in the middle of the night. We climbed up on top of school buildings and stretched out on our backs to look at the stars. We sat on piers at midnight, letting our feet drag through icy salt water, or built bonfires on the beaches, staring across the water at the lights of Seattle. I thought up mad plans involving hundreds of people in my plots to make everyone wear *E.T. Lives* buttons or protest against the school administration.

I squinted at my friends when they talked about crushes,

watched in baffled amazement as they paired off. I could not imagine the mechanics of a crush. Was it something that people chose to do, or something that just happened? What did it feel like? Was it even real at all? I was engaged in an enormous project to seek out the simple things I had missed as a child, sleeping while everyone else played. Those years left me with a sort of irregular innocence, an everlasting inability to look at other people; instead, I looked at the sky, or the trees, or my own shoes. It wasn't because I was ashamed; I never felt ugly, even as the scars accumulated. The doctors had often conveyed that my body was fascinating, that the disease was less a burden than a prize. The disjunction between their attitude and the taunting of my peers was difficult to sort out, so I didn't think about it.

As a general principle, I could not figure out the point of romance—not even the sham varieties—and decided that it must be something akin to a bodily function. Perhaps I was missing an essential enzyme that would allow me to become overly fond of my friends. It didn't really matter, because crushes seemed to lead to physical contact, and by the middle of my adolescence I did not want anyone to look at me or touch me without permission.

One day this kid named Joseph called and said he had six tickets to see the Cure's *Kiss Me Kiss Me Kiss Me* concert. He had to fly out to see his grandparents and wouldn't be back until the day of the show; would I track down everyone who was going, since he had run out of time? I said yes; it was the type of thing I did routinely. I drove all over the county to locate people and arrange the time to meet at the ferry terminal. My friends said the person who bought the tickets was cute; they raised their eyebrows and asked if I was going on a date. I laughed at the thought. Why

would anyone want to date me? And even in a mad alternate uni-
verse where that might be the case, wouldn't such things require
my consent? I had no plans to date anyone. Ever.

But at some point during the concert, this person I had never
taken much notice of grabbed my hand. I looked down in shock—
my fingers were entwined with his and it was odd. What could he
be thinking? I looked away and pretended that nothing was happening. Surely he would stop if I ignored the whole thing. From
what I could gather from novels, suitors expected their advances
to be accepted or rebuffed. If I just held my silence maybe the
whole thing would evaporate.

Then one day we were in a park, sitting on a balancing beam
watching our friends do tricks on skateboards. Joseph kept
moving closer and closer; I grew nervous and started to laugh. He
moved his face close to mine and looked directly into my eyes.
His expression was serious and determined, and by then I was
laughing so hard my nose was wriggling from the exertion. I wondered why he didn't stop, could not imagine why he kept pressing
in, and he leaned in and kissed me.

This, then, was what all the other kids knew: Kissing was fun.
It didn't matter if you wanted to ahead of time, or liked the
person. This was deeply interesting information. He kept kissing
me and, after a few days, it seemed fairly clear that I had a
boyfriend. He stroked my face and hands and eventually my neck,
coaxing me to let him see what I kept covered up. He touched my
scars and said that I was beautiful.

I didn't believe him, wasn't even too sure that I liked him. But
physical pleasure is a tricky thing, and soon something was radiating out from the middle of my body, quickening my pulse.
Romance made sense finally; it was a wholesome, healthy hobby.

My scars faded to silver and it looked like my body was covered with drops of rain.

One hot summer day I decided to go to Mt. Rainier to visit a friend who was working in the lodge. My car was in the shop, so I borrowed my mother's new white Chevrolet Sprint. Joseph, Elizabeth, and a kid named Christopher came along.

The road to the mountain winds through second-growth forests and abandoned lumber towns, along rivers, and up into a protected national forest. Even though you can see the mountain from anywhere within 200 miles on a clear day, you never know that you are climbing up until your ears pop—the view of the incline is completely cut off by the dense trees. On the way we stopped at Narada Falls, admiring the water tumbling down the canyon, and talked about theosophy.

We stopped at Longmire and I spread out an old white table-cloth printed with roses for our picnic and we sat in the sun eating sandwiches and fruit, surrounded by goldenrod, butter-cups, fleabane, columbine, thistle, and yarrow. I told my friends the stories I knew about the early development of the area, how the springs were considered medicinal and people would ride up on horses to take restorative cures. The afflicted paid twelve dollars for passage and eight dollars per week for treatment—an enormous sum of money at the time. I wondered if the beauty of the place comforted some of the terminally ill as they passed through.

After lunch we drove further up toward the glacier and parked next to the visitor's center at a place called Paradise. We wandered around, staring down at meadows filled with wild-flowers, then up at the dome of the mountain towering and white against a blazing blue sky. The gift shop had pamphlets in twenty different languages, flocked toy deer, volcanic ash bulbs, and ice cream bars.

Our friend met us at the service entrance to the lodge and led us down back hallways, through little-used rooms and secret passages, up the rear staircases and along more passages, into a guest room, and we looked out over the vista of the park. He told us ghost stories and we shivered over the hidden history of the old building. It looked more like *The Shining* than I was ready to contemplate, and I was glad that I was not old enough to spend the summer working away from home. When it was time for him to go back to work we realized that it was getting late. We said goodbye and set off down the mountain.

Joseph had put a tape in the car stereo but it was broken and wouldn't play. We stopped at a rest stop; the first orange of an imminent sunset came down sideways through the trees, illuminating green leaves and gray bark. Christopher talked about being in love with a girl called Pell-Mell. Elizabeth was worried about the upcoming school year; she had always been a good student. We were all planning to apply to colleges in the state and debated which one might be the best choice. I stretched and said it was time to get back on the road.

In the car, Joseph started to read a novel. Christopher and Elizabeth fell asleep, their heads resting against the windows. I looked in the rearview mirror at my sleeping friends and smiled. Then I noticed a big white car tailgating and started to look for a place to pull off and let it pass. The sun had not gone down yet and the evening sky was saturated with streaming colors—pinks, reds—reflecting on billowing cloud formations.

I was still smiling when I realized that a car traveling in the opposite direction was crossing the double yellow lines into our lane—it was so close I could see the driver's dark hair curling at her shoulders. I tried to throw the wheel, but her car was coming too fast. When the other car hit us I felt the impact fling my body forward, and back, then my car spun around and the white car following hit us too, head-on.

The world went silent.

I was crushed and blinded and surrounded by a searing white light. I could not see or move and my mouth wouldn't cooperate with my thoughts. It was like waking up after general anesthesia. Was I dreaming? Was this another surgery? No, it was an accident. We had a car accident. People have car accidents. Don't panic, just be practical and check on the others. I pushed against the static light and asked if everyone was OK; there was no response.

I repeated, "Is everyone OK?"

Christopher groaned.

"Are *you* OK?" I asked. He didn't answer and I shouted at him, "Look at Elizabeth, is she alive?"

His voice was thick when he replied: "Her forehead is gone."

I felt around the front seat for Joseph, but he wasn't there. Someone came to the window and told me an ambulance was on the way, told me to be calm.

"Where is the boy who was in the front seat?" I asked.

There was silence and then a heavy sigh. The voice replied that he had been pulled out of the car, not to worry, he was fine. I reached up to touch my head and it was wet. I asked the person at the window to call my parents and repeated the number over and over.

Rescue vehicles came. I could see a little bit, although everything was stained red and purple. I couldn't really move

enough to turn around and look at the backseat, and someone
kept talking to me every time I tried. A woman in a beige shirt
with long, bleach-blond feathered hair reached in to stroke my
arm. She made note of my parents' number and promised to
call. Then she was gone and in her place was a teenage kid
younger than us with a wispy moustache, his hair in a mullet,
wearing a Metallica shirt. He was the sort of kid who would have
threatened to beat us up in school, but he reached inside the
car and held my hand and kept me talking, gently turning my
face away from the backseat whenever I tried to look. I asked if
he could call my parents. He wrote the number on the back of
his hand.

A paramedic explained that they would have to take Elizabeth
out first because she was unconscious. He asked if she was pregnant and I was so surprised I laughed. Couldn't he tell we were
slightly bohemian geeks, honors students, *good* kids? Then I wondered what sort of injury she might have to make her appear
pregnant, and fell silent.

He asked where we were hurt.

"I'm fine. *Fine*. No pain," I replied.

Christopher said, "I can't feel my legs."

The rescue crew pulled Elizabeth out through the hatchback,
then Christopher, twisting their bodies past the cooler and the
remnants of our lunch. Someone wrapped my head in the rose-
print tablecloth we had used for the picnic, explaining that I had
to be protected from the shattered glass. The paramedics hacked
and sawed the car open to reach me. The seat had buckled,
impaling me against the steering wheel, and my legs were trapped
under the engine. It took three men to wrench and yank me out
of the wreckage.

Months later I saw state patrol photographs of the three cars jumbled to one side of the highway. The two that hit us were huge and old—dented, but not destroyed. The photographs show the entire front end of my mother's car compacted into a sheet of twisted metal. Tires were ripped off, the roof collapsed, the front seats torn from their runners. The pictures show blood smeared across the seats, dripping down the outside of the car. The tablecloth used to cover my head was abandoned on top, soaked with blood.

When we were all lying on stretchers in the ditch I heard Christopher arguing that he didn't want them to cut his pants off. The paramedics did anyway. Then they cut off my shirt, sacrificing all our gentle modesty to a ditch on a highway.

The ambulance crews said they were taking the boys to an army hospital nearby. Elizabeth had not woken up and my head was taped to a board. I was worried that she would die without last rites and asked if we could go to a Catholic hospital together. The sun had set but the summer sky was still bright. I stared up, the brilliant sparkle of concussion making it look like the clouds were dancing. It felt like my heart was providing the music, thumping and skipping with an ominous beat.

Someone covered me with a sheet and then we were in the ambulance and I started to shake so hard my head rattled against the board, hair caught in tape tearing away from my scalp.

Elizabeth woke up as we passed the neon sign for an ice skating rink in Spanaway. "What happened?" she asked.

"Don't worry, we had an accident. You are going to be fine."

"Where is my mom?"

"We'll be at the hospital soon, it will all be OK. I love you. Please rest and feel better."

She didn't say anything else during the ride.

The hospital staff rushed to take Elizabeth away. They left me in an examination room. Every twenty minutes or so a new doctor or nurse would show up to talk about what happened.

"You were the driver? Were you drinking, using drugs? Were your passengers wearing seat belts?"

"No. I've never, ever had alcohol or drugs," I replied. "Of course we were wearing seat belts. Will you please call my parents?"

The police came, then more doctors, all asking the same questions, ignoring the blood I could feel trickling down the side of my head. I heard them muttering about teenage drivers just beyond the pale blue curtain surrounding the gurney, and my body started to shake even more. My bladder felt like it might explode but the nurses shook their heads no when I asked to get up to use the rest room. A lab technician jerked my arm to the side, rubbed a cotton swab across a bloody elbow, and jabbed over and over until she was able to get enough blood to verify my claim that I had not been using drugs.

I had been strapped down with tape and belts for five hours when a doctor finally came to attend to me.

He said my eyelid had been slashed open, and that he would need to fix that first. As he stitched the wound, he told me he had seen Elizabeth. "She is in surgery now. I don't think she'll make it." I shuddered and he yanked thread through my skin. "The boy in the backseat certainly will not live. Let that be a lesson to you next time you want to go joyriding," he said, as he tied off the knot and walked out of the room.

I stared up at the ceiling, trying to count the tiles, but I couldn't see that far without my glasses and my right eye had swollen shut. The world was still pulsing and red and my head felt broken. I wanted my mother. Instead, Elizabeth's mother showed up next to the gurney.

She patted my hand, still strapped at my side. "It will be fine," she said. "I've called your mom. Just try to stay calm. We don't know where the boys are, but we're trying to figure it out."

It must have been another hour before my mother arrived; the hospital was far away from our home. I was still strapped to the board but her face appeared above me.

"I'm sorry I wrecked your car," I said.

For the first time ever, I saw my mother cry.

With my mother standing sentinel, a nurse finally pulled the tape off my head and unbound my arms. She listened as I asked for a rest room, but replied, "Honey, I don't think you are going to make it that far. I'll get you a bedpan."

"Oh, please, let me walk," I said, but she left and came back with the pan. She was right; I could not even sit up without help. My mother and the nurse propped me as I urinated, eyes closed against the indignity of needing help with such an intimate chore.

The medical staff looked at my torso—bruised from hip to throat—listened to my chest, then started to hurry through tests. My heart had been damaged by the impact.

They rolled me onto a different gurney and sent me upstairs to intensive care. I was hooked up to monitors and an IV and told to stay in bed. The nurse was named Jessie James; he called me "sweetheart" and used a warm damp washcloth to clean the congealed blood off my face and neck.

When my parents and the medical staff left, I swung my legs over the side of the bed and hobbled over to the mirror on the wall. I saw for the first time what I could not feel: My face had

been smashed—eyelid lacerated, cheekbone fractured, jaw dislo-
cated. I put my hand on my chest and swayed. The heart monitor
raised an alarm and nurses came rushing in to put me back in
bed, telling me not to worry, just to rest.

Further examination revealed that my collarbone, ribs, and
pelvis were fractured. I had a head injury. I had torn cartilage,
muscles, and tendons in my back and arms. I had major nerve
injuries in my legs, arms, and face. My hearing was damaged and
I had lost my sense of smell. But this constellation of trauma did
not hurt. I could not feel anything.

I wanted to know if my friends were OK, but nobody knew
the complete facts. They told me Joseph had gone through the
windshield head first, his face slamming against the torn metal of
the engine block. They told me that Elizabeth had indeed lost her
forehead, along with forty percent of her intestines. They told me
that Christopher's spine was broken, torn in half.

The nurses knew that I did not want drugs, but one distracted me while another covertly added a narcotic to my IV
drip. Sleep intervened.

induction

Byron showed up at the hospital at about nine in the morning. He had packed one of my old flight bags with a change of clothes, makeup, and the shoes he had inadvertently taken home the night before. I told him that I was on track for surgery. He was astonished and asked, "Are you sure?" In the ten years we had lived together I had never willingly gone along with even basic medical testing without extraordinary research and the fretful interrogation of multiple experts. Byron was certain that I would try to wriggle out of it somehow, but this time I didn't see any other option if the doctors were correct.

Maybe Byron had a point. What if I had allowed myself to be sucked into a quagmire of mainstream medicine? What if there were alternative approaches, wacky diets, some option other than surgery? We couldn't figure out how to research this, since there was no Internet access in the hospital.

I opened the bag and pulled out the makeup. This was not an act of vanity; several layers of concealer, powder, and lipstick provide protection from the sun, make it less likely that I will develop more cancer on my face. Even the weak light coming through windows can be a dangerous level of exposure.

Another hour passed before I decided to call out for a second opinion. I picked up the phone to call one of my own doctors. He listened to the description of the symptoms and then asked in a worried voice, "Where are you? Not in your hometown?" When I told him which hospital I was in, he said, "Oh, that's just fine! They are the best in the city. You can absolutely trust them."

When the surgeon showed up with a pamphlet describing the procedure, we listened attentively and asked many questions. I made eye contact with him, ascertained that he would remain in the room throughout the operation, clarified stray points of concern related to my other surgeries, and told jokes that made he and the resident laugh. Growing up sick demands a set of unique skills. If I had not been able to impress the doctors with my winsome ways, I would have rescheduled for a different doctor on a different day.

The surgeon was still trying to figure out the extent of my internal abdominal scars and said, "So, remind me: You have had one appendicitis surgery, one peritonitis surgery, and two C-sections—"

I interrupted to say, "No. I delivered my first child the normal way."

After the accident I stopped cutting my hair and sat through high school classes with my head bowed, letting a sheaf of tangled fine blond locks slide forward, obscuring the scar. At first I told my mother I would cut it when everyone was out of the hospital, but that day passed along with a hundred other milestones, and still I could not sit down for a haircut. There was no reason behind this choice, just a quivering sense of dread. Even after the injuries healed I let my hair grow, streaming down my back untended, tufts catching in zippers and car windows.

I stayed up every night watching reruns of *Bewitched*, sitting in the living room with my dog in my lap, avoiding sleep for fear of nightmares. As a small child, I had been devoted to the show and taught myself to wiggle my nose just like Samantha, but now found that I could not repeat the trick with all the fresh injuries to my face. Specialists offered plastic surgery to fix the shoddy, uneven work of the ER doctor, but I refused.

The driver who caused the accident had no insurance; she declared bankruptcy and claimed she had no memory of what happened. The driver of the car behind us did the same. I was not allowed to talk to the friends who had been in the accident because our attorneys felt silence was necessary until the cases were settled. The insurance companies were fighting; everyone wanted us to file a product-liability suit against the car company.

I would never have guessed that the lawsuits could drag on for five long years of subpoenas and depositions and skirmishes, featuring my testimony as the only witness. Although no one died, two of my friends would need multiple surgeries over the course of a decade. One would never walk again. At the time, all I knew for sure was that we all had glass working up through deep wounds, slivering out of our skin at unexpected moments.

I hallucinated blood dripping down the walls if I let my eyes stray away from the television or the printed page. I could not smell anything real; instead, I smelled and tasted blood every minute of every day. If I sat in the front seat during a car ride, my whole body flinched each time I saw a car in the opposing lane. If someone tried to toss a towel or a ring of keys for me to catch, I had flashbacks of the impact, the white, brilliant explosion of glass and bones breaking.

Attorneys pressed me to submit to a mental health evaluation to establish my value as a witness. The psychiatrist said that I had an organic head injury with classic depressive characteristics, along with clinical post-traumatic stress disorder. Then he said that I was afflicted with survivor's guilt and magical thinking—that it was unsound that I believed in coincidences and contingencies, rituals and repetition. Apparently the tricks and habits learned during seventeen arduous years of incapacity were aspects of mental disorders. But if that was true, what else should I have done? What the doctor called "aberrant" looked like necessary skills to me. He wanted me to take drugs, but I rolled my eyes. The last thing I needed was a new set of disorders to keep track of, tend, and nurture. I walked out of his office and never went to therapy again.

My parents said that I had to start driving right away, but I could not face the prospect of my rusty old car. When they tried to coax me into driving my father's truck, I stood in the middle of the driveway with no shoes on, shaking my head. Finally, I screamed at them that I would never drive again, then ran into the house. They left, and a few hours later came home with an old Volvo station wagon, solid and huge, with good, strong seat belts.

I didn't want the gift but also did not want to be stuck in the forest with nothing but my dog and my memories.

I set off on long trips around the Northwest, driving away from the forest, through the mountain passes, across the desert, watching my headlights illuminate an empty landscape. More than anything I wanted to turn the wheel away from the road, send the car over a cliff or off a high bridge, but if my friends had any hope of getting settlements, I had to stay alive long enough to testify.

The sweatshirt cut off my body by the paramedics was tucked in my hope chest. When my arm came out of a cast at the end of the year, I pulled out the shirt and started to stitch the ragged pieces back together.

I spent the summer after high school graduation wandering around wearing peacock-shaped sunglasses and vintage gray silk pajamas, waiting to move away for college. One day I was sitting in court talking to my attorney when he introduced me to another one of his clients, a boy named Paul. He had freckles and short blond hair and he wouldn't tell me why he was there. When Paul was called to the bench, the judge charged him with communicating with a minor for immoral purposes. I laughed out loud and the attorney shushed me. The boy asked for a ride home and invited me to go ice-skating.

He told me stories about stealing boats and playing chicken with the state ferries. He introduced me to his friends, who had all spent time in prison or mental hospitals; several had been interviewed in connection with murder investigations. He asked permission to kiss me and I said yes. He taught me how to shoot a gun.

I was too weak to use a revolver, but it did not take long to learn how to hold a semiautomatic. The metal object felt good in my hand: heavy and lethal. Within a few days I could place five bullets in a fist-sized target at fifty yards without pausing, the immense power of each shot blasting up my hand and riding the track of injury, ruined nerves pulsing with sensation.

It was difficult to settle into a new life as a university student. Every weekend I drove home to stay with my parents and see my friends. Paul worked in a lumber yard and on his days off we went on more long road trips, driving around the state, staying at roadside hotels with broken neon signs. Late in the autumn term, the joints of my arms and hands started to swell. I went to see one of my own doctors but he decided I was simply homesick.

Four months passed and I felt worse each day. I started to lose weight rapidly, felt dizzy and sleepy all the time. When my hair started to fall out again, I drove back to the peninsula to ask the doctor for more tests. I wondered if I might be having complications from the accident or the stomach surgeries—the doctors had warned me that the scar tissue could cause serious problems at any point over the years. Or perhaps I had developed a different variety of cancer. I had a hunch that this might be the case and it was a welcome thought. Death represented respite, and death by disease would be an easy exit. It wouldn't be my fault. I could just give up, go away.

The doctor had treated some of my extraneous symptoms as far back as the first cancer surgery. He knew my history, knew my family, and was generally regarded as an excellent physician. When I started to describe the symptoms, he frowned over my chart and shrugged. "These are ordinary complications of pregnancy," he said.

Pregnancy? "When you did tests last time, I was told they were all clear," I said.

He tossed the chart down on the counter and washed his hands. "That has happened to a few people recently."

I walked out of the clinic in a state of confusion. Having a child was impossible. I had been assured that I was not capable of it. I was too sick, too poor, and too young.

It would have been practical to terminate the pregnancy had the doctor given me the test results in a timely fashion; it would have been safer never to have gotten pregnant in the first place. It was theoretically improbable that I would have a good outcome, but my entire life up to that point had been pathological. Teenage pregnancy didn't rate. The most disturbing problem was figuring out how to tell my parents; aside from the colossal health risk, I was the first person in the family to go to college, and my parents were proud of me. I snuck home in the middle of the night and left a note on their bathroom mirror.

Of course the doctor had been overly optimistic. The symptoms might have mimicked a standard pregnancy at some point, but most women have morning sickness and assorted discomforts —some minor, some severe—that are always within a well-defined category. I had a violent rash on my forearms and a red mark the shape of a butterfly on my face. I could not gain weight, even after putting myself on a special protein diet. My joints were tender and hot, and I started to have muscle spasms that sent me to bed for days. I went back to the doctor and asked for more tests.

I was eating scrambled eggs and working on an essay for school when the nurse called with the results of the blood work. She paused between each fact, careful to make sure I understood. I sat, watching the eggs congeal, and then picked up a pen to write notes on the back of my schoolwork. There was no mistaking what this meant. The lab tests verified that I had systemic lupus.

The diagnosis had been on the periphery for five years, never quite acknowledged but always a risk. My body, damaged beyond the limit of what can be tolerated, had finally conceded the game. My immune system had started to attack and destroy otherwise healthy tissue. The nurse said the doctor had declined to see me again. I would need to find specialists.

I did some research. *Lupus* is a Latin term implying that the disease ravages patients like a hungry wolf. The books said that drugs and treatments had advanced in the last few decades but categorized juvenile onset lupus as a potentially terminal diagnosis. Pregnancy was not advised, even when patients are nominally healthy, because the antibodies can cross the placenta and attack the baby directly. That is, if the mother can carry a pregnancy at all: late-term miscarriage is common.

The only reason I hadn't been on significant painkillers during the previous months was my stubborn refusal. As far as the doctors were concerned, I was still in danger of developing lung cancer and should be having frequent diagnostic tests. The surgeries for skin cancer had slowed but not stopped. My injuries and abdominal scars were, as the doctors told me, *extremely* serious. People hovered over me in clinic waiting rooms, trying to impress me with their facts and stories. They frowned and said that it was too late for an abortion, but that I should get used to the idea of not having a baby. They said that I should listen, pay attention, follow orders. They said that I might die.

Paul took me to the hospital the first time the muscle spasms in my legs proved incapacitating. He sat next to the bed, head bowed. He was frightened and suddenly thrust into a form of adulthood that must have been deeply repellent: a prospective teenage father with a girlfriend and baby who might not survive the ordeal. He decided to join the military to earn more money. By then I was too ill to argue against the plan. I understood the logic and had no claim on his time. He wanted to do the right thing, to be a man, even if that meant never seeing his child; I wanted someone to hold me. I closed my eyes and nodded. What difference would it make if he left? I was used to being alone within illness. The world recedes and other people are just phantoms, whether they are in the room or halfway across the world.

It looked like the doctors were going to take over again, and I fixated on the idea that I must deliver without any surgical interventions. I didn't want them to cut me.

Before, my choices had been to either succumb or survive. I was just a kid adrift in an impervious system, and I never had the chance to decide on a course of treatment, negotiate my care, pick and choose. This time I wanted to make my own decisions about my body and the baby. There was not a doctor within a hundred miles of my home who would agree to take my case.

Everything I did after this point—from leaving college and moving in with my parents, to extensive medical testing three times a week requiring a 200-mile round-trip commute for appointments in a high-risk clinic at the teaching hospital—was in the interests of the child. Even my seemingly quixotic determination not to deliver by Caesarean section was based on valid health concerns; surgery lends no greater security to the infant born to someone with my diagnosis, and it may increase complications.

My pregnancy didn't involve dreaming, wondering, picking out toys. I was not even healthy enough to shop for maternity clothes; I wore my father's T-shirts and castoffs from my mother's friends. I drove the Volvo vast distances for appoint-

ments and sat in waiting rooms reading medical textbooks and
alternative health guidebooks.

The tests revealed I was having a girl and I decided to name her
after my great-grandmother. She had divorced her husband
decades before it was socially acceptable, raised a raucous group of
kids on her own, and took a job as a welder in the naval shipyard
during World War II. Family legend claims that when the men came
back the other women went home, but my great-grandmother kept
showing up every day. The bosses were so flummoxed they never
managed to fire her. I figured my daughter would need that kind of
strength. All of my thoughts were devoted to protecting the baby
and keeping her in my womb as long as possible.

Lying in my childhood bedroom I stared at pink walls,
butterfly-print curtains, shelves lined with the stuffed animals
people had sent after the surgeries, cabinets containing dolls and
glass shoes and stacks of books. I stroked my little dog—by then so
ancient he could no longer see or hear—and he squirmed with joy
to have me home again. Casper slept on my pillow each night as
muscle spasms shivered down my frame; I could not roll on my
side or even turn my head.

Pain crushed my lungs like an immovable 400-pound
weight. Esophageal spasms seized my throat. I had almost no sensation at all in my arms except a dull tingling. I felt like my skin
wanted to crawl off my skeleton. When I could fall asleep, I awoke
over and over again scratching so viciously that I had long, deep,
purple bruises down my arms and legs.

Laboratory tests indicated that treatment with steroids was
compulsory, but I refused the drugs because they would only ease
my pain, not protect the child I was carrying. They might even
damage the infant, limit her potential and cognitive abilities.

The doctors in the high-risk clinic were baffled by the case—not just my perplexing array of complications and disorders, but also by my level of resistance to their suggestions. They had never met a disabled, working-class, pregnant teenage girl with long blond hair and a preposterous voice who could debate them word-for-word on any technical statement.

I refused to sign their forms, insisting that they seek my informed consent for even the smallest procedure. When they told me the clinic's doctors would rotate, I refused to change my lead physician. When they sent students to attend to me, I sent them away. It wasn't because I was afraid: An entire lifetime of medical drama had left me incapable of feeling fear. I could tolerate great pain without protest. I had no hope, but plenty of anger, and acted with fierce determination.

The doctors warned that my body might kill the baby and I consented to amniocentesis to determine if her lungs were mature enough to force a delivery. They poked a needle in my belly to siphon off the fluid required for the test. She wasn't ready, and I defied the doctors by carrying her longer.

At that point I was in a full lupus flare and had been refusing to deliver the baby for six solid weeks. The muscle spasms increased. My expanding uterus inexorably shredded all the scar tissue from earlier surgeries and I curled into a ball around the pain. I was ordered to go on bed rest, but the doctors didn't know that I was driving myself to the appointments, weak fingers gripping the steering wheel of the Volvo. Eventually I was too tired and ill to drive across the bridges, around the bays, and thread my way through traffic, so I took the ferry instead, sleeping in the back of the car for the hour-long ride.

The baby grew bigger and pressed against my pelvis, which had been fractured in the accident. The symptoms were wearing me down. I was subjected to twenty-four-hour urine collection tests to monitor my kidneys, which were failing. I had to consent to an induction.

I held a pen in my clumsy, numb, injured right hand to write the instructions for my funeral.

The nurse hooked me up to an IV and monitors and I waited for twenty-seven hours for drugs to stimulate my uterus. Finally, a doctor took a tool that looked like a knitting needle, shoved it inside of me, and broke the amniotic sac. Fluid rushed out of my body and I turned my face away in embarrassment just as a precipitous labor started. The contractions on the monitor were continuous, with no breaks, not even for seconds, and an ultrasound showed that the baby was in an awkward position. For the first time in my life, I demanded pain relief.

The anesthesiologist thought that starting the epidural would be easy—*roll on your side, don't breathe, here we go*—but he could not puncture my spine. I felt the first, second, third, fourth, and fifth attempt, holding still as the contractions wrenched my body. I stared at the window frame and contrived to trace the shape of the ship canal to the south of the hospital with my mind. The doctor was mumbling and pale by the sixth puncture, when he managed to start the line. He patted my leg and asked, "Did anyone ever mention that you have scoliosis?"

I shook my head and gritted my teeth. The epidural would not do much more than make my legs numb.

Labor was an inexorable, inescapable, *real* pain that could not be ignored; it was beyond my capacity to understand. It was horrible and beautiful and nothing like being cut or examined. It was nothing like appendicitis, broken bones, or cancer. It was something beyond all reason. My body moved and contracted and tensed and relaxed for a different purpose, for something new and peculiar.

In my memories I am alone, but in fact a dozen relatives and friends were in the waiting room. My mother and Angie were with me, standing with their backs against the wall, distressed to watch me taking such a huge risk. They had both loved me through too many other crises to be happy with my deliberate decision to have a child.

My baby burst into the world with a splash of blood, fist-first and facing the wrong direction, ripping me asunder. She had huge eyes and a strong wail. The specialists were sure she would be in crisis and they took her to be evaluated before showing her to me. But she was perfect, without flaw, without any trace of the auto-immune disorder that could have crossed the placenta or even the myriad deficits of normal infants.

I sat with the baby for a few minutes, touching her small face and nestling her against my shoulder. She held her head up, looking from side to side, new to the world and imperious.

I had met my goal: I had created a vibrant little person who was not damaged by steroids or incipient disease. No scalpel had interrupted her journey. But I kept bleeding for several hours, and a junior doctor sent me back to the surgical suite. My mother held the baby and I was wheeled away, protesting. In the hall I saw Angie crying and talking fast on a pay phone, trying to convince someone to donate blood.

Drugged with an incomplete epidural and high on adrenaline, my body going into shock from loss of blood, there was very little I could do to protect myself.

I was alone with a doctor who would not listen as I insisted that the blood was coming from the tear, not from my womb. He proceeded to do an internal exam, his hands ripping my fresh wound open even further. Blood spurted wildly and hit the doctor in the face. If I could have moved my legs I would have kicked him in the head. I wanted to cry, I wanted my baby, I wanted to be rescued, but the only weapon at my disposal was the threat of a malpractice suit. My voice was steady, clear, and cold when I said, "I specifically decline consent for this procedure. Take your hands out of my body."

That got his attention and he turned away, brushing the blood from his cheeks.

My body started to shake violently, just like after the car accident. I demanded a new doctor, who confirmed that the injury was external and then stitched the brutally torn skin and ruptured artery.

I didn't cry—not then.

Nursing the baby in my own childhood bedroom, I realized that the illness was ebbing away. Months passed and the pain disappeared; I had feeling in my arms again, and was strong enough to play with my little child. I went back to college, started a part-time job, and filled my days with work and caring for the baby.

My little dog faded as the baby grew. His world had contracted to include only a blanket in the corner; he could not find the door to go outside. He was no longer strong enough to jump up and sleep on my pillow. The skin under his matted white fur had turned purple. I didn't know what to do, felt that acting to end his suffering would be like murdering my best friend. He was the only creature of any species who loved me without any complicated expectations, but he was nineteen years old. His life was drawing to an end, and it seemed selfish to ignore his suffering. He must have known about the baby, must have felt the displacement. One day I put him in the car and drove to the vet and held him in my lap as he was injected with a lethal drug.

Back at home I sat with his blanket and cried all the tears of an entire fractured childhood.

danger

Byron worked on his laptop while I looked through a week-old newspaper. The only reading materials in the visitor's lounge were decrepit copies of *Sunset*, *Reader's Digest*, and a sticky three-year-old *People* magazine. *What a wasted day*, I thought to myself.

There was no point in sending Byron out for a book. I wouldn't be able to concentrate; I couldn't even focus on the television. Later in the day I would be recovering from surgery, but for now there was nothing to do, no preparations to be made. My job was simply to wait.

I wasn't nervous; my mind had slipped into its old familiar and serene pattern: empty of critical thought, unable to feel fear. I slipped an extra gown on backwards, tied the ribbon enclosures, and asked Byron if he wanted to go for a walk.

Two days earlier we had both been productive and busy. Now we were adrift, without work or parenting responsibilities to occupy our time. I wondered what the children were doing; it was time for lunch recess at school and I pictured the boy on the jungle gym, the girl laughing with friends on the game fields.

After a few minutes of indecision, we set off down the long corridors and peeked in different wards. There were separate sections for people with heart disorders, people with head injuries, the elderly and dying. We searched for the maternity ward, hoping for a glass wall and babies in rows like in the movies, but when we found it there was just a security door with a buzzer.

One building of the hospital was connected to another by a sky bridge and we walked across to find ourselves in a large glass atrium. An art show had been set up with dozens of photographs of one scene, a time-stop sequence of a vacant lot. The images showed an old woman arriving with a grocery cart. She opened up a bag and started to scatter crumbs, and then she was surrounded by an enormous flock of birds. They ate the bread and flew off again. The old woman walked away with her cart.

I stared at the photographs, idly curious about why they had been chosen to decorate this vacant, echoing, purposeless room. Walking over to the window, I looked down at the view of a gray dirty alley filled with dumpsters. A cloud passed in front of the sun, shooting shadows across the reflecting glass walls of an office building across the street. I watched a dented red van drive up and park next to the dumpster, and a brown squirrel climb a drain pipe. I sighed.

One sunny day I left my daughter with her grandmother for a few hours and drove to Olympia to see a band called Some Velvet Sidewalk. My waist-length hair was held back with a chiffon scarf, and I was wearing an electric-blue mini-dress. There was a boy named Gareth sitting next to me.

Driving across the Tacoma Narrows Bridge, Mt. Rainier on the horizon and sailboats far below, I reached out to change the radio station and Gareth smacked my hand away. Without a pause my hand reacted, curling into a fist, and my arm jerked back, up, and with vicious force connected with his face. Without analysis or planning, without losing control of the car hurtling at fifty miles per hour over a high bridge, I had hit back as hard as possible. He held both hands to his face. His voice was muffled, blood was trickling through his fingers, and he started to cry. "You broke my nose," he said.

Some hair had flown across my face and I tucked it back under the scarf. "You shouldn't have touched me," I replied.

The diseases and treatments rendered me tough and defiant and adept at controlling the superficial and visible portions of life; the head injury left me nervous, twitchy, with a flinching hyper-awareness of my surroundings and my own lack of skills. I knew how to wear outlandish clothing, take care of a baby, write an essay, and shoot a gun. But I did not know how to look at other people and did not care to try.

However, if someone wanted to kiss me, that was reason enough to proceed; there was no notion of preference or attraction. I didn't care what other people looked like, how they had grown up, or who they were connected to—I just wanted physical pleasure without emotional involvement. It was immaterial if my date was the fiancée of a murder suspect or my boyfriend's best friend.

Before, I had thought my friends represented a happy idyll, but after having the baby I now saw something below the surface. Out of a group of thirty people, only six moved away to college; three of us stumbled home again within a year. I was still taking classes, but living with my parents. Most of my friends didn't have plans to leave town.

Looking around, I recognized that every single person I knew was damaged in some way. There were girls sticking their fingers down their throats or carving their arms with razor blades, boys taking massive quantities of drugs. Some people were dabbling in domestic drama, beating each other up as a form of entertainment. Presumably there were other sorts of people nearby, but the ones who showed up in front of me had long before been devastated by sundry incursions on their lives. My friends had been inevitably corrupted by the reality of life in a hard, poor town and the dangers that befall children when their mothers are not vigilant in protecting them, body and soul. Violence was just a regular part of life, no different than a hundred other small details of the landscape.

On Mother's Day I was sitting in my parents' living room watching television while my daughter napped. I heard a loud bang, then a thump, and something hit the side of the house. I looked out the front window and saw a fifteen-year-old neighbor named Adam lying flat out on his driveway, something long and metallic on the ground next to him, flecks of red and white and gray all around his recumbent figure. Doors were opening up and down the street; adults were looking from their porches, kids were walking toward the source of the noise. Adam's father ran out, the screen door banging behind him, and knelt beside his son, then put his arms under the shoulders and lifted the body. The head was gone, blown away by a self-inflicted shotgun blast. Later that evening, after the police and ambulance crews left, Adam's dad unspooled a garden hose and stood in the yard for hours, sending jets of water across the blood-spattered gravel, fragments of bone tumbling into the ditch.

One of the kids I knew opened his dad's gun cabinet, loaded two revolvers, and put them both in his mouth, pulling the triggers simultaneously. A girl drove her car into the side of a grocery store. Someone took the ferry and never arrived on the other side. Other people jumped off the Tacoma Narrows Bridge; one climbed up in the spires and dove from the very top without checking the direction of the wind. She landed in the middle of a road choked with cars, the ruined mess of her body flattened and smeared by drivers who did not know what fell from the sky. Traffic was stopped for seven hours as road crews scraped the remains into plastic bags.

The suicides seemed both inevitable and logical, and I do not recall anyone railing against the squalid waste of these young lives.

People were not even particularly shocked by murders. As I grew up, there were three serial killers stalking people in the Northwest; one targeted prostitutes, one preyed on little boys, another seemed to have a broader appetite. The newspapers dutifully reported the deaths, a parade of torture and sexual mutilation and fear, and our mothers cautioned us to be careful, avoid strangers, trust only the people we knew.

But that advice was not always helpful. I was in my bedroom studying when I heard another shot, this time from the house behind ours. It was late, nearly two in the morning, and the shot was followed by sirens and a knock at the door. I peered out my window; it was a cop. He wanted to know if I had seen anything, heard anything, but I said no. The next day someone told me that a seventeen-year-old named Russ had dressed in camouflage, stood over his parents' bed, held a shotgun over one face and then the next, asking politely why they had beaten and humiliated him—why exactly they thought they should live. He directed them to beg for mercy. Then he shot his father in the face.

There were more stories; it never seemed to end. One day I was trying to read the newspaper with the baby on my lap. She patted my face with her chubby little hands, cooing. I held her tight and walked around the house, trying to figure out how we could afford to move away. I thought that if I was deliberate and practiced at being an adult the way some people join a sports team, maybe we could have at least a facsimile of a decent life.

When several of my friends were raped by someone we all knew, this kid named Anthony turned up with a gun; he made various threats and the culprit decided to move to another state. Anthony was honorable, smart, amusing, and strong. He liked me and I figured he represented safety. I could already protect myself, but if I joined ranks with someone equally powerful I would be invincible.

We rented a basement apartment from a man who lived in the top level of the house. He kept four Doberman guard dogs and the place was structured like a compound with eight-foot-high wire fences. Whenever we were home the dogs peered in the windows, checking on our safety. I went to school, Anthony went to work, and when she wasn't being looked after by her grand-mother, my daughter toddled around, playing peek-a-boo with the dogs.

One night we argued about money. There was never enough and Anthony was working too hard; he said that I was selfish to stay in school when we needed more income. I didn't really care what he thought, and lacked the wisdom to keep that information to myself. The quarrel ended with a 9mm handgun held at my right temple. Anthony was not shaking with rage, flushed with power, blustering and roiling with emotion; he was steady and determined, the barrel of the gun pressed against my skin an admonition, a malediction, and I neither doubted his intent nor his ability and willingness to act.

If he could provide a defense he would argue, *But you had a knife*, and this is true. I had a sharp and lethal knife pressed to his stomach—and knew how to use it. Even if I couldn't survive this fight, I could inflict damage.

We had both been wounded by our short, fast lives and the inescapable events that brought us to this particular moment, standing in the shabby white kitchen of a dank basement apart-ment, dirty dishes on the counter, school papers scattered everywhere. I looked at his round, young face, at his brown eyes deciding when he would pull the trigger, and remembered all the other moments of rage, the other fights I had won or lost.

I thought, *This can be the end of all the fighting; it would be so easy*. Simply being alive had been such a terrible war of attrition. I had survived by a narrow margin, and I could have opted to do so many other things with this hard-won victory, but I had chosen this boy and this moment. I had used up all of myself and was still no more than a mile from my childhood home; I was on the far side of the same forest and my daughter was asleep in the next room.

"Put it down," I said quietly, and continued looking into the madness of his eyes until they fluttered, closed, and he stepped away.

I never saw Anthony again after that night. His sister came to help him pack up his things and I waited in the yard, a light mist fogging my glasses, until they were gone. People tell me he did well in the end; I hear that he married and moved to Alaska.

My own ticket out of town arrived in the form of a settlement check from the accident big enough to pay university tuition, put my daughter in day care, and rent a room near campus.

I'm still drawn to the grown-up children of violence, the people who keep secrets and show off lies—but I keep them at a safe distance and politely decline to play. I have a strict and repressive code of conduct for myself, and I will not fight, nor debate, nor will I even speak to people who might cause me to fall down again, to follow that reckless, thoughtless slide into the rage.

Those of us who grew up fighting know each other without telling these stories, we can smell it maybe, or perhaps see it in the way a hand rests on a table. Maybe we hold our bodies differently, maybe the message crosses our faces before we even know that we have given the secret away. I do not consciously try to convey information with my body, but I've never been harassed by strangers. When I walk through a large crowd people move swiftly out of my way.

calculated risk

An hour before surgery, a nurse came to ask me to take off my
jewelry and makeup. My fingers were swollen, but I tugged at my
rings until they came away, leaving deep grooves in their place. I
took off my silver earrings and wiped off my lipstick. The nurse
pointed at the yarn tied to my wrist.

Several weeks before I had gone to a party for a baby who was
not yet born. The midwife directed a series of rituals to protect
the mother and infant during birth, and at the end all the girls
and women in the room were bound, wrist to wrist, to offer soli-
darity and power for the journey. We were instructed to wear the
bracelet until it broke naturally. I do not enjoy group cere-
monies, but when your body is stripped down to a basic survival

level there isn't much left to believe in. If knowing that we were wearing yarn around our wrists would help this woman as she gave birth, then I would wear the yarn. I didn't want to cut the bracelet off, so I pulled it slowly across my hand and used it to tie up my jewelry.

Byron walked next to the gurney as I was wheeled down to the surgical suite. When the attendant parked me in the waiting area, I sat up and squinted around the room, although I couldn't see much without my glasses. The anesthesiologist showed up with a clipboard; he would have liked more details about my history, but I couldn't do better than a vague memory of adverse reactions. I did remember to point out that my jaw joints have no cartilage and asked him to be gentle while inserting the tube down my throat.

When it was time to go in to the surgery I turned to Byron. "Do I have lipstick on my teeth?"

"Let me see." He squinted as I pulled back my lips. "No, your teeth are completely prepared for this experience."

"OK, thanks. By the way, that can be my epitaph."

"What?" He looked confused. "Her teeth were prepared?"

"No. It should read, *Do I have lipstick on my teeth?*"

Byron laughed and kissed the top of my head and then I was wheeled away, leaving him helpless in the waiting room. The last time I had surgery he was able to stay with me throughout the procedure; that was the day our son was born.

One evening after I moved away from the peninsula to live near the university campus, I was studying in my room while my daughter stayed with her grandparents for the night. A housemate knocked on the door. I didn't really know him or anyone in the house very well. The contrast between my life and theirs was too extreme.

It annoyed me when I reflected on the fact that most students seemed to think there would always be time for whatever they wanted to accomplish. There was no time for me in the sense that my peers seemed to anticipate, future years filled with conversation, creativity, making music, and traveling. There wasn't even time in the sense that another mother might hope for, with privacy, space to think, breathe, and sleep. I imagined that finding time was like opening a birthday present—something special and rare, something you didn't expect to receive and can use in whatever way you like—while the expectation of a long life is even more generous, a warranty against disappointment, a tonic to soothe anxiety.

Nothing like that existed for me; there were only absolute notions of ethical integrity and a small child to take care of. But even as I enjoyed her company, I knew that I had to work harder to give her a chance for a decent life. I could not take a year off or study abroad, because I needed health insurance and that meant a job. There were bills to pay, a career to choose. When I finished college, Elizabeth insisted on giving me part of her accident settlement to pay for graduate school; it felt like a blood oath, like I had to stay in school not just for myself but for all of us.

I boxed up the fancy clothes, cut off my long hair, and picked a new life. The goal was to stop being special, intriguing, different. I wanted to be a stable, middle-class professional, and I knew how to select that outfit even if it looked awkward on me. It would have been nice to see time as negotiable. But that was a fantasy, so instead I did my schoolwork.

The housemate who knocked on my door was named Byron and he apologized for bothering me. He was having an asthma attack and needed to go to the emergency room. There were no busses that late at night and nobody else in the house was willing to give him a ride. "Of course," I said.

When we arrived at the hospital he opened the car door and thanked me; he said that he would walk home after the treatment. "In the middle of the night? Wheezing?" I asked. "No, I'll wait for you."

Months later he gave me a ride to the hospital for the final session of radioactive isotopes. We went to see a matinee of *Malcolm X*. Was that a date? I still have no idea. Eventually, after I rented a cabin and set up a household with another friend, Byron drifted in and never left.

My earlier relationships had featured high drama, without real reward. Byron played with my daughter and read drafts of my masters thesis even though the topic bored him. He was there for all the good and exciting events but also the mundane and tedious. I was suspicious, waiting for the inevitable crisis, not ready to care too much about someone who would leave. But instead of trauma there was school, a daughter to raise, and a nice fellow who never wandered away. Instead of observing or reacting, I was actually participating in my own life in a way that had never before been possible. If this was love, it seemed to be about reciprocity and disciplined attention to details.

I was twenty-five years old when I decided to have another baby.

Byron was doing doctoral research, my daughter was in kindergarten, and I had been working in disability activism, implementing federal civil-rights laws in state government agencies. Working on hard projects that required intense focus left little room for worry.

The remission from disease seemed sustainable; the major cancer had been gone for over a decade, the skin cancer had tapered off, and there had been no discernible problems with my immune system for six years. I followed the basic rules, stayed out of the sun, went to the doctor for check-ups, and started to believe that I was safe. There were limitations and some areas of permanent disability, but I was no longer sick. I never even caught viruses. The only worrisome reminder of the past was a startle reflex; loud noises and flying objects made me jump. The diseases were just memories, a series of macabre stories that I could sometimes rearrange into raffish anecdotes to amuse colleagues and clients. I went to work, did my job, and had fun taking care of my family.

I looked at the academic calendar and holiday schedule, calculated when it would be most convenient for the baby to be born, and marked the proposed date of conception on the calendar. Then Byron and I took out a license and got married. Two days later, exactly as planned, we conceived a child.

My body, so uncooperative in the past, was able to carry a pregnancy. I ate the correct proportion of fruits, vegetables, and protein foods. The baby grew according to program, and I asked for genetic screenings that put my fetus under intense scrutiny to identify potential defects. We learned that we were going to have a boy, that his spine and brain were developing at the correct pace, that he would probably be taller than his father. We also learned that the placenta covered my cervix.

This was a mechanical complication, a risk in every pregnancy, not something related to my prior history. We were assured by the perinatologist and the obstetrician that the placenta would move up with the expanding uterus. The vast majority of similar cases noticed in the first trimester correct themselves by the second trimester. I hired a midwife and planned to do a homebirth, or if that became impossible, at least she would help me during a hospital birth.

But my placenta did not move, and the only available treatment—suggested not only by the midwife but also by the high-risk specialists—was to visualize change. I sat around the house imagining the placenta creeping upward.

After several weeks I started to bleed. There wasn't much to do except continue the mental exercise and stay in bed. Even after the bleeding stopped, the pregnancy started to feel more like a miscarriage than a viable baby. I was allowed to pick my daughter up from school, make snacks, and go to medical appointments, but other than those tasks, I was required to remain in bed and focus on only positive thoughts. I was not supposed to worry, and specifically was not supposed to retain in my mind the fact that a stubborn placenta previa which does not move so much as a millimeter is quite likely a placenta accreta, which in turn means a risk of death to the mother and baby. It also, without exception, requires a Caesarean section followed by a radical hysterectomy. I didn't want to be cut again, and definitely did not want to lose my uterus. I had already lost enough of my body through the years.

There was no rousing of a community to offer solace and assistance. There was no discernible community of any kind; I had devoted a lot of effort to making us look like respectable middle-class people with careers, systematically choosing clothing and haircuts for everyone in the house, and this had proven more alienating than I could have anticipated. We looked like we didn't need help, and therefore did not receive it. The few friends I had pulled away when I was confined to bed rest. The midwife had been paid in full through barter—for months Byron and I had watched her troubled foster kids when she needed help—but when the situation became complicated, her commitment wavered.

In the second half of the pregnancy I was at a medical appointment when I started to bleed again. I didn't tell the doctor what was happening because I knew that I would not be allowed to leave. My daughter was at school, Byron was out of phone reach, and I needed to pick her up.

I drove myself, bleeding, from the hospital to the school and tried to convince one of the trustworthy parents to help me. She agreed in a desultory fashion to watch my child for the afternoon but made it clear that she would do no more. I gave my little girl a kiss and drove myself to a different county to check into a Catholic hospital.

It was a calculated risk—I knew that if I was able to keep the pregnancy I would be admitted for the duration. I also knew that an HMO would not be polite about sterilization. I suspected, and still believe, that they would have taken my uterus rather than risk the expense of additional pregnancies.

Catholic hospitals are not allowed to offer information about birth control unless it is solicited by the patient, and even then employees may opt out of the discussion because of their faith. I gambled that my atheist soul—and my uterus—would be safer with a crucifix over the bed.

However, without consulting me, the doctors held a special session with experts from several fields, took a vote, and sent someone off to the archdiocese with a report about my interesting history. Despite the mandates of their faith-based hospital, the doctors sought and received special dispensation to sterilize me after the baby was born. They must have thought it was a favor; they certainly did not understand that they were insulting me on a philosophical and political level when they shared the news.

When I stared at them with no expression, then coldly inquired if their suggestion was sympathetic with the doctrine of the Church, the doctors tried to reassure me that I was not committing a sin. When I started to expound on the interesting implications of mixing up religion and medical malpractice, they quickly withdrew the offer and assigned a priest to come and visit me each day.

For the next five weeks I was on full bed rest, restricted to lounging on my left side, but I resisted the routines of the place and would not wear a gown or crawl into bed. Resting on top of the hospital blanket, dressed to make a quick escape, I pulled a blanket Byron brought from home over my head and put my hands over my ears. I did not feel sick, or injured, or weak, and I had never been compelled to rest except during the illnesses. Trapped in bed, I could not stop thinking about the early tests, procedures, treatments, surgeries; my small body broken down to the most basic individual parts, a child younger than my own daughter, trapped in a nightmare that I could never wake up from. Hospitals and doctors had taken everything away, stripped me down like an old car at my uncle's wrecking yard. I took their lists of rules and built something unexpected, something that repudiated everything that had happened to my body: a family, the most essential element of society. This was my choice, and I had done everything possible to make sure the baby was safe. The new complication had nothing to do with my past, or the baby's intrinsic health, and it would be better for both of us if I stopped worrying.

I was too tired to read and tried to listen to the radio, but BBC news reports were all about the slaughter in East Timor; this distracted me in a way not conducive to rest. I turned off the radio and closed my eyes, letting my mind revert to old habits, calculating and cataloguing.

Byron had classes, work, and a six-year-old little girl to take care of alone. We had absolutely no support from anyone. Not a single friend came to our aid and our parents were too far away. The midwife decided I was likely going to die and went on a road trip without following the protocol of her profession and asking another midwife to take over.

My daughter says she learned to read during this time; she remembers driving up the highway and seeing signs pointing to the left for the zoo and the right for the hospital and asking if they could please go to the zoo. She played at the foot of the bed for hours as Byron studied and nurses dropped in with popsicles and kind words.

The baby was high and breech and rarely moved, as though he understood the danger waiting for him. One morning more than a month before my due date, he flipped and his head engaged with the placenta. Blood streamed out from between my legs and the doctors rushed me into surgery.

I told the doctors that epidural anesthesia does not work on my body, but they didn't listen as each successive puncture of my spine failed. Finally, after the seventh attempt, they thought the medication had taken effect and they cut me quickly, a line straight down from my belly button. I could feel the incision and had to hold still as the scalpel ripped through layers of skin and muscle.

My voice was crisp when I said, "I can feel this."

"Some women feel a tugging, pulling, wetness. That is normal," the doctor slashing me open replied.

"I feel you cutting me," I said, in the wintry voice that always appears when I am pushed beyond tolerance.

"No, it is just . . ." the doctor started, and then Byron was yelling and I could not hear anything.

Some women say that they forget the pain of childbirth, but I remember what it felt like to be sliced open without anesthesia. I remember seeing blood smeared across surgical dressings, remember the look of fear on the face of the anesthesiologist when he realized I was telling the truth. I passed out after a shot that did not dull the pain but did allow me to lose consciousness, waking intermittently to a slantwise view of the surgical suite's white walls.

I woke up in the recovery room, grabbed the rails, and pulled myself to a sitting position to see Byron holding our son. The baby was five weeks premature, with raspy lungs, making a mewling sound. I pulled aside the receiving blanket to look at his tiny body, skeletal and quivering, then covered him up again.

The nurse showed me a chart with smiling faces turning to frowns and asked me to assign a one-to-ten value to my pain. I refused, and when she said I would not be allowed to leave recovery, I replied flatly, "My pain is zero. I feel splendid."

The doctors took the baby away for evaluation. Back in the room, the television was on, *Apollo 13* playing silently on the small screen.

A nurse came to take my temperature. "Where is my baby?" I asked.

"He needs to stay in intensive care," she replied.

"Can I go there?"

"No. Your surgery was too complicated. They did a classical incision, which means you will need more recovery time." She walked out of the room.

I turned to Byron, slumped in a chair, twisting his hair around shaking fingers. When he looked up his eyes were red and swollen from crying. "The blood was everywhere. It looked like a can of paint had been splashed all over the room," he said. "I thought I had lost you."

If I had ever wondered about the mechanics of love, this moment erased all doubt. Love can take many forms, yet some varieties wither under the strain of daily life. Byron, like my mother, would never give up on me, and respect and affection had grown into a full-fledged sentimentality. Pain and love surged through my body, one overwhelming the other.

"Don't worry about me. I'm *fine*. Please go get the baby. I don't care what you have to sign. Bring him back to me."

Byron left the room and I switched off the television and closed my eyes. I must have slept, and then Byron was there with my son. I cradled him in my arms and looked down at his small, perfect face. He had no expression; his eyes were closed. I could hear the sighing of his lungs.

I put the baby inside my gown, held him tight, and let my body be his incubator.

singing

My arms were strapped down and the drugs entered my system. I fell asleep and dreamed of houses with arched ceilings and bulbous blue light fixtures, flagstone floors, hidden passages, and an old lady lying on a couch, dying of cancer.

I woke up to see a man spinning around and around on a stool next to my gurney. He was wearing a blanket over his scrubs. When he heard me cough, he stopped spinning, discarded the blanket, and congratulated me on the weak rattle I had produced.

"Do you want me to cough more or less? I can do either," I said, craning my neck around to see a clock. "How much longer do you need me to stay here and what can I do to speed up my departure?"

He laughed and sent a message out to tell Byron that I was fine.

Back in my room I pulled down the blankets. Five small

bandages informed me that I must have had the laparoscopy, though it had taken about three times longer than the doctor had predicted. Byron showed up and told me some facts about the surgery that I could not track through the fog of pain. The narrative included information about scraping scar tissue off my liver and abdominal wall.

More blood tests were ordered and a technician came into the room pushing a cart, with cotton balls and rolls of adhesive in tidy rows, glass vials rattling. He asked which arm would be best and I looked down. Both were covered in bruises, but the right arm was also host to the intravenous line. I reluctantly held out my left arm. The lab tech whistled a tune I could not place and pushed up the sleeve of my gown. He saw the lower portion of my tattoo, pushed the gown higher, and exclaimed, "Wow—that is amazing. Did it hurt?"

I tugged the gown back down. "No."

After the technician left, Byron asked, "Do you want me to call anyone?"

I thought about it for a minute. "I don't want my mother to worry."

Byron sighed. "OK, but what about your friends?"

"Why?"

"Because they love you and want to know what is going on."

"How do I know that for sure?"

"What about the bicycle? The parties? The letters, postcards, and e-mail? The fact that your friends will go hundreds of miles and whole continents out of their way to visit?"

"No," I replied. "I don't want anyone to see me like this."

After my son was born, it took an entire year to recover from the surgery and for the baby to catch up. The consequences of prematurity are both harsh and subtle; the baby needed to be held and nursed constantly, required a pristine silence in the house at all times. As I paced the floors holding my sensitive child, I had hours and months to decide what to do next.

Eight years of working in nonprofits and government agencies had taught me that community does not always occur automatically, out of proximity or need. Sometimes an administrative initiative is required. That concept could be applied to the experiences I had as a young parent; no institutions existed that could have helped me, connected me to others in a real way. I started with one far-fetched idea, and set out to create something new for the disenfranchised parents of the world: a series of projects that would offer solace to people who, for whatever reason, could not find friends. I had no reason to think that my idiosyncratic notions would be helpful to other people, but the projects consumed my time and years passed in a blur of work and taking care of children. Running my own business meant that I could once again wear the clothes that had been packed away years before; the middle-class costume hadn't worked anyway.

One day I met a woman who was in a radical chorus. She was organizing a fundraiser and wondered if I would come and set up a table to let people know about the work I was doing. The group she belonged to performed political folk music at protests and demonstrations, events and festivals. They believed that everyone should make music, make as much noise as possible. They rejected the notion of standards, although they practiced each week. There were classically trained musicians mixed with people who had never learned to carry a tune, ones who had recording contracts sitting next to others who had never bought an album in their lives. The motto of the group was "Subversion through Friendliness" and they claimed to be "the chorus that is more fun to be in than listen to."

The first time I saw them perform they stood in a row, dressed in tattered pirate costumes. They opened their mouths and sang energetically, voices rising. It was not always a magnificent sound, but it was honest and real and they all looked like they were having a scandalously good time.

Byron and my daughter joined the group, attended the practices, performed, and the other members became our friends. I watched them joke and laugh and sing, and invited them to use my house for practice. They sat in my living room in a circle, drinking tea, learning how to harmonize. I watched from the doorway to the kitchen and wondered if I could join in.

When the doctors opened my neck to remove the cancer, they explained that my vocal cords would probably be amputated. If they could avoid that, everything would be moved to the side, pinned out of the way during the surgery. The procedure damaged my superior laryngeal nerve and left my voice weak and prone to failure. I had never been a loud person, but after the surgery I became even more reticent, because there is no voice to spare, and because I sound like a demented eight-year old. When I am talking, my voice is erratic and often fades in the middle of sentences; no amount of training can ever restore full control. I never learned to sing because I thought that I did not have the physical ability to do so.

But this group of people didn't care about perfection, about striking a pose of professionalism. I listened to them week after week, memorizing the songs, and started singing with the kids when we went out on walks. It was true that I could not sustain a song from start to finish, but if I wasn't trying to sing *well*, then I wasn't wasting what little voice I had available.

During one session I sat down in the circle, picked up a songbook, and tentatively joined in. At first the words were just a whisper, but soon I was raising my voice along with the others, a reverberation of sensation shivering down my neck and throat and through my abdomen.

The chorus sang at a union rally. We performed "Banks of Marble," "Coal Tattoo," and a song with the refrain, "Our lives shall not be sweated from birth until life closes / Hearts starve as well as bodies; give us bread, but give us roses."

Our house was derelict when we bought it, with a backyard that featured flashing shards of broken glass and three stolen cars. All the windows were boarded up, and the kitchen ceiling was riven with rot. Over the years we had restored the place one room at a time, scraping bumper stickers off door frames, sanding floors, revealing features we hadn't noticed when we signed the mortgage papers. Chorus members helped us with some of the projects, shifting a dozen ancient washing machines out of the basement, painting rooms, hauling in truckloads of dirt from a distant farm. When we laid out the garden we found that the soil was littered with the remains of animals burned in a barn fire, teeth and jawbones and pelvises crusted with dark clammy earth. My son was certain they were dinosaur bones and we arranged them in a circle around the new herb garden.

The basement of the house has nearly 800 square feet of dry storage, with phantasmagorical blue and yellow patterned linoleum from the late 1960s. I filled the space with racks and the vintage dresses I had been collecting for years, garish polyester shifts from the 1970s alongside square-dancing outfits that crowded against formal wear from earlier decades. There are racks devoted to faux fur coats, and others hosting sequined circle skirts decorated with paintings of cheerful holiday scenes. Several dressers hold the undergarments and accessories that go with the outfits, and shelves are burdened with intricately designed handbags that match every conceivable combination of outfits. Trunks contain the pieces I let the children use as costumes, a seemingly endless supply of pinafores and spaceman outfits, hats and ball gowns, swords and scabbards. The amount of clothing is so vast there is always something new to look at when I walk down the stairs. I invited the chorus to use my costume boxes for the events.

There were concerts, performances, and parties. One summer we went on a road trip to perform in another state and twenty chorus members stayed at my house the night before. We were up most of the night laughing and making food. After the others went to sleep I walked through crowded rooms, looking down at my sleeping friends, bemused. I had been alive for twenty-nine years and didn't think that there was any point lamenting the past; the life I had created was satisfying. I had in fact achieved adulthood with all the trappings, including a family and a real job and a few good friends. But community was something I gave other people through my work; I never thought I would find it for myself.

Apparently everything had just been out of sequence. I was experiencing what I had missed during the cancer years: spontaneity and casual joy as a member of a group, without violence or terror on the margins.

The next day everyone assembled in front of my house in a caravan of rickety, clanking old cars and vans, most without seat belts—and if there had been, nobody was interested in wearing them. I rented a big white car and everyone who rode with me was tightly buckled.

After we had been singing together for a year I was talking to a chorus member named Dwayne and we realized we had grown up in the same place, that he was the boy who worked at the record store near my high school. We talked about our homes on the peninsula, and how much we missed the forest. He had two former guard dogs that had been rescued from abusive homes, and they were vicious enough that Dwayne had on occasion hired attorneys to represent them. The dogs had bitten half a dozen chorus members, and I would not let them anywhere near my children. But when we were alone together the dogs sat close to me, resting their muzzles in my lap, staring up at me with mournful eyes.

The chorus went to a house party to raise money for a legal defense fund. We sang "Broceros" and "Rote Zora" and a Utah Phillips song that included the refrain, "All the agonies you suffer / You can end with one good whack / Stiffen up, you orn'ry duffer / And dump the bosses off your back!"

I was wearing a green and pink floral print square-dancing dress, and held my right arm tight against my body, angling myself away from the group for fear they might jostle into it. On icy mornings, or when the seasons changed, my injured arm always got numb, and sometimes there was a flash along the nerve that runs between the smallest finger and the elbow. Years of work and too much time in front of the computer had made the situation progressively worse, and earlier that week the wrist gave way, flopping uselessly at the end of an arm surging with pain. I had sought medical advice, but the doctors shook their heads and told me that there was no hope; they said the damage was irreversible, that not even surgery could help.

I had always been too poor and too skeptical to try alternative medicine, but now that Byron and I were earning enough to cover the bills and leave a surplus, I wandered among my chorus friends soliciting their advice on treatments. People suggested various holistic approaches, and I held a pen with awkward, numb fingers to take notes.

I went to see a chiropractor. He listened to my complicated history and said, "I feel intimidated." He told me it was clear I could survive anything, but that it was no longer necessary. He said that I needed to learn not to be stoic.

Later that week I went to see an acupuncturist. She listened to my story, then said I was used to being an archetype, either dismally sick or miraculously cured. She said that something in between would be better.

She put needles in my arms and feet and in the middle of my forehead. She used a cup and flame to treat my back, enormous dark bruises blooming on my pale skin, darker over each scar. She kept asking if the procedure hurt, but it didn't feel like anything. The bruises reached from my tailbone to my hairline, black and blue and speckled. She looked at the marks and said, "You have bad chi."

One of the chorus members was a qualified massage therapist. Ana Helena manipulated my arm and watched my face and then sharply directed me to come back into my body. I was startled and realized that everything had gone gray; I had let my mind wander free, had become the good patient who can take any procedure or pain without flinching. She said that it was good that I could feel pleasure, be decadent, and have fun, but that I needed to learn to feel pain too. She said I had to learn to feel the pain if I ever wanted to get better.

Ana Helena offered to work on my jaw. Surgeons and specialists had assured me that the joint would never recover, that the cartilage was simply gone. I hadn't been able to yawn or eat an apple in twenty years, and figured it couldn't hurt to try to get some more movement, to make the muscles more limber even if the bone was intractable. She put her fingers on my face and pressed on all the points of injury. She kneaded the skin in front of my ears, pressed down on the old scar on my eyelid, rubbed the point at which my cheekbone was fractured. I heard a popping sound inside my head and the world seemed to dissolve for a moment.

After the massage I dressed and drove home. Something was different. What was happening? It took several hours to realize what was wrong: I could *smell*. For the first time since the accident twelve years earlier, my brain was exercising a lost sense. It was not a complete recovery, more like a twenty-percent cure, but I could pick up the scent of pine needles in the yard, a passing car with a bad muffler, candles someone had burned in the house. It was a completely foreign feeling, and the mental files telling me the meaning of scents opened slowly.

Weekly acupuncture appointments and massage started to help my arm. I began to feel warmer. Instead of cold and stiff, my joints felt like rubber bands after just weeks of treatments.

The chorus sang at a police accountability rally. There were police with automatic rifles lined up on the sidewalk and on top of buildings staring at us as we sang "Hard Travelin'" and "Kill for Peace" and a slew of songs about police brutality.

One day a chorus friend named Marisa was helping me move boxes in the basement. She asked, "What do you identify as?" She might have been asking a general philosophical question or inquiring about my career; she might have been asking, *Are you straight or what*? I wasn't sure exactly what she wanted to know, but I replied, reflexively, "Nothing."

Marisa raised her eyebrows. "What would you say if pressed?"

I turned away to sort a stack of clothing and shrugged: "Nothing."

The truth is too complicated. How can anyone answer the question? What makes an activity an identity? I did not feel that the children, the career, or my dating habits defined me. It didn't matter what I had chosen, or what I had accomplished.

My primary identity is found in my body, in the scars, in the injuries and injustice and disease and decay. My genetic code conveys the simple truth that I'm a freak; no other information about me is relevant. But nobody can see that now. The clothes and family and job act as refraction, creating an illusion to distract people from seeing the truth.

Moving further into the basement, I found a box containing my old toys. Here were Nestor and Lucy, waiting to be found. Polaroid photos showed happy times in between surgeries, swimming in lakes, playing at the beach. The *E.T.* scrapbook fell open to the pages of hospital bracelets, and I rubbed a finger across the wrinkled plastic. I picked up a small pink satin dress that I had worn at age three, and found the tiny metal baton with my name etched on the side. My double vision had not prevented me from marching in parades with other little girls, sequined tiaras pinned to our hair, twirling batons, our mothers walking next to us smiling with pride.

Another box held all the letters anyone had ever written to me and several hundred I had mailed, then later retrieved. There were piles of photographs from high school, all of my friends caught forever glaring out from under awkward haircuts. The next box had the file from the lawsuits, with photographs of the car and my injuries clamped in a binder with pounds of paperwork, the depositions and reports and settlement details warping slightly from dampness. Another box contained X-rays and medical charts, stacks of paper detailing my years of incapacity.

When Marisa left I took the medical records and legal documents out to the backyard, built a fire, and burnt them all, sending smoke and ash up into the night sky.

The chorus performed sea shanties at a zine release party. Byron took a turn at the microphone and presented his doctoral thesis as a performance piece; it is a mathematical opus titled *Structuring Instruction Sets with Higher Order Functions.* He was accompanied by modern dancers interpreting the work. Many audience members sat in baffled silence, but all the chorus members were doubled over, laughing.

After the performance I went to the kitchen to get a glass of water. Someone asked me to open a jar but I couldn't do it; I found Dwayne in the living room, held out the jar with one hand, and turned my other palm up, explaining, "I'm weak."

He stroked his finger down the length of my arm. "You are not weak," he said, "you are strong." I shuddered. He was right, but I didn't want to be strong in that way, not even if it was attractive and desirable. I wanted to be like my friends, riding their bicycles madly

down big hills, stripping naked and running into rivers, singing
without wondering if their voices would disappear entirely.

A girl named Raki wandered by and heard me say, "I have no
problem with the big important things. But I still don't know how
to hug my friends."

She stopped and clapped her hands together. "I know exactly
what you mean! Hugging can be the hardest thing. What you need
is lessons."

I laughed and nodded. Raki asked for a volunteer from the
crowd and a girl named Anna Ruby stepped forward to show how
you hold your arms to indicate willingness, how you place them
around another person. Raki made Anna Ruby pose in different
ways to demonstrate the cues that people use to show that a hug is
not wanted, or that it is time to let go. Then she asked me to
practice. I put my arms around Anna Ruby and closed my eyes.
The lesson might have been offered as a joke, but I wanted more
than just a perfunctory ability to open my arms. I held on to
Anna Ruby, smelling the rosemary oil in her hair, feeling the
edge of a patch on her sweatshirt. The tenderness of the embrace
spread warmth to my cold, battered joints.

Over the next few weeks the warmth in my joints turned to
heat. I looked in the mirror and saw that my face was round; the
remission from lupus seemed to be ending. The sweet drowning
sensation of disease was radiating outward from somewhere deep
in my body. I stared at my face in the mirror and wondered if
eleven years of relative health was over.

I asked the chorus to practice somewhere else because I was
ill. When they did not see me as frequently I no longer heard
about the parties and excursions. One day someone left a huge

bag of vitamins and supplements worth hundreds of dollars in front of the door, with an unsigned note wishing me well.

Every night Byron held me as I lay curled up, arms crossed, trying to remain calm and imagine myself well. I tried to believe that my children, husband, home, work, and friends made life worth conquering the disease again. I tried to care that one-third of my life had been conducted with little trace of disease—this was surely an accomplishment—but the abomination of the illness distorted everything, and I stared up at the ship-lathe walls of my bedroom in the eaves. Something must have triggered my immune system. I had painted the room myself; did the exposure to chemicals hurt me? Could it be the new ability to smell—could the recovery of a lost sense shock me sick? Could the new treatments be the problem, snapping and cracking and sucking toxins and terror up through a corporeal host? Or perhaps it was the singing: Maybe the vibration had shaken something loose.

Byron urged me to go to the hospital, but I knew what they would say. Everything was restricted. The rules regarding my health are extremely specific: Take these drugs, go to bed, surrender to reality.

The alternative health practitioners offered another set of goals and objectives. They were helping me, but the appointments and attention made me feel bone weary, reminded me of being a special little girl in yet another hospital.

Languishing in bed as my thirty-first birthday approached, I decided that I wanted a symbolic break from the illness, the disease identity, the doctors, and all the rest of it. But what could I do? The need for safety was so deeply ingrained, and connected to physical limitations, it was hard to conceive what freedom looked like. I was stuck not only in the bed, but also in the city, tied down by medical treatments, caught in a net of obligations to other people. Even the work that I had ardently pursued was another tether on my body that required daily attention. I thought that instead of following the rules, perhaps I should follow the example of the chorus and stage a mutiny against my own body. I had learned to sing and embrace my friends, both of which had once seemed impossible.

Any other time I might have made a list of trivial events, catalogued the contents of bookshelves, tried to distract myself from the stupefaction of a dissolving body. But this time I pulled out a journal and started to list the things I could not do: ride a bicycle, travel, eat unusual food, walk outside in the sunlight, and dozens of lesser restrictions that controlled my daily life. Some were valid, but there were many others, orphaned attitudes and postures that had no business lingering. Even though my adult teeth grew in white and strong, I was still holding a hand across my mouth when I laughed, unable to break the habit of a little girl with rotten teeth.

Byron drove me around the city to different restaurants and we ate things I would have politely declined in the past. Food had often been dangerous, a source of pain. During the years without a sense of smell, I couldn't taste much; my palate could only differentiate between sweet and salty. There were no nuances, no subtleties, and the material I put in my mouth was just fuel. But now everything I ate was a discovery; even a bagel and coffee from a cheap and dirty storefront were exquisite. The taste of Afghani chickpeas, Senegalese plantains, spicy Indian curries, and dozens of other new dishes were explosions in my mouth, heady and invigorating.

The idea of being on a bicycle, exposed and without protection except for a thin plastic helmet, was anathema: dangerous and absurd. My injured arm was not strong enough, and even if I could ride I would look foolish flitting about in my sequined skirts. But several of the chorus members were bicycle mechanics, and one day I went to the shop where they worked to look at a row of old bikes. My friend Erin pulled down a black Triumph, and I looked at her strong arms, covered in tattoos down to each knuckle. I wanted to ask what the images meant, ask why she decorated her body, but I inquired about modifying the bike instead. She offered to customize the handlebars, seat, and brakes to accommodate my injuries. I paid the bill and went home, confused. Could it be that easy to do something impossible?

One day I had to go across town while Byron was using the car. It was easy to take a bus on the errand, but I picked up the phone and called a taxi. For the first time ever, I left the seat belt unbuckled. My palms were sweaty; riding in a car without a seat belt was idiotic. But speeding through the city streets, I rubbed my damp hands on my skirt and kept my face resolutely turned toward the window.

That night I bought a ticket to go to Italy; this would be the first time I had traveled without the children or a work commitment. Printing the itinerary confirmation, I felt like I was breaching an invisible film that had always existed between me and real life.

I went to bed and dreamed of a heart pierced with a dagger, of swallows flying across a low hill by the sea. I woke up and made an appointment to get a tattoo of that image that would stretch from my shoulder to elbow. I did it quickly before a doctor or my mother could point out the risks and the impossible stupidity of the decision.

When I walked into the tattoo studio the guy at the counter looked me up and down. "Bet you five dollars she faints!" he shouted over his shoulder to the person who would do the work on my arm.

I stared at him until the smile faded from his face, then replied, "Bet you $500 I won't even flinch."

When the needles entered my skin I looked down at the hands gouging a deliberate design over erratic scars. It definitely felt like something, but it wasn't pain—I could tell the difference. I laughed.

I learned to ride my bicycle, wobbling along side streets dressed in polyester tennis dresses, wearing a huge black helmet. Perhaps the alternative health treatments were the source of the recovery, or maybe I would have healed without intervention, but within a few weeks the illness had retreated and my injured arm was warm, strong, repaired. I rode through the city smelling everything, the good and the bad, the lovely and the rotten.

make-believe

I asked to get up and use the rest room and the nurse seemed surprised but went along with the plan. When I got back in bed, shrugging aside all helping hands, the nurse strapped a blood pressure cuff to my arm and attached it to machinery behind the left side of the bed. Then she placed my IV on the right side, blocking access to the telephone, and plugged it into the wall at ground level behind a dresser. She pulled up the sheets and yanked what looked like large white tubes onto my legs and plugged them into a machine that in turn inflated the garments. The machine was incredibly loud, and the suctioning pressure—in and out, in and out—made all the small hairs on my body stand on end.

I was entirely trapped and tied down. The machines on both arms were bad enough, but the things on my legs were cumbersome and sweaty and scary. I couldn't bend my legs or adjust my position in the bed.

"Excuse me, but what are these?" I asked.

"They help your blood circulate so you don't get clots," she replied.

"This is really unpleasant. I would rather not have them; I'm willing to get up and walk to keep the blood circulating. Can you take them off?"

The nurse shook her head and started to fuss with the IV pole. I tried to shift in the bed, tried to think of a better argument.

I was too distracted to ask what she was doing as she injected my IV with something. I shouldn't have had to worry; my chart clearly stated that I did not want pain relief and can't take morphine or codeine because I have an allergic reaction and go manic—all pain is enhanced to dizzying effect and I just want to get up and pace.

The nurse left, a drug flooded my veins, and I started to writhe. I raised the bed to a full sitting position, gripped the metal rails, and bit my lips as the muscles in my neck and back started to spasm. I turned to Byron and said, "I'm freaking out. What did they put in the IV?" He walked to the door and looked at the chart hanging on the wall outside. "Morphine."

"I will not be able to handle this. I need these socks off. Can you go find someone who will agree to let me get up?"

He left the room and I sat waiting, trying to resist the urge to slam my head against the IV pole. He came back to say that the nurse and resident had both said no.

"Fine," I replied. "Please close the door and draw the curtain."

After the room was secure I said, "Take these infernal things off my legs."

Byron laughed and stripped the socks off. "Now what?" he asked.

"Hide them in the cupboard and put the extra blanket over them."

I unplugged the power source of the IV and swung my legs over the side of the bed. Byron slid wooly socks on my cold feet and held my hand as I stood up; I shook off his support and shuffled out of the room.

The first time I walked past the nurses' station the person on duty frowned at me. The second time I rounded the hallway someone asked if I might feel more comfortable resting. By the third time they were used to me and distracted by other patients.

When I was a child, my mother coaxed me to get up and walk after surgeries, chided me when I refused to take a drink of water. She knew that the trick to getting out of the hospital is to simply *get out of bed*. She held my elbow as I walked through the corridors, one foot slapping down after the other, fresh wounds still crusty with blood. She brought my stuffed animals and books, but she never let me believe the lie that the hospital was a place to recover health. As far as she was concerned, the only way to get better was to get home again, and in this she was absolutely correct. I would have walked home if I could have put my own shoes on.

Back in the room I drank all the water in the decanter provided and used the phone to call downstairs for copious amounts of cranberry juice and ginger ale. My throat ached and I ordered milkshakes to soothe the inflammation. My face was covered with strips of adhesive debris and I rustled up some alcohol swabs to clean the mess. Technicians stopped by the room for more botched blood draws, new bruises fanning across my elbows and hands.

Most people with January birthdays will admit that the event is grim and dour. The weather is miserable, people are tired and often sick with seasonal viruses, and if anyone remembers to give birthday gifts it most often takes the form of an extra note on a Christmas card. My own birthday is still notable as the anniversary of the first cancer surgery.

When I was younger I was mainly irritated by the fact that I didn't get enough presents. I used to be angry at the casual disregard I received on my special day, used to buy myself special treats. After I grew up I decided to throw myself parties. At first there were just a handful of people sitting in the living room; the next year there were dozens. Within a few years there were hundreds of people milling about, spilling into the yard, swarms of small children running around, adults of all description laughing and talking to each other. But even with so many people crammed into the house, I always feel alone in January. The memories are singular and cannot be shared.

My medical routine dictates a minimum number of checkups and I avoid them until January, deliberately letting despair stack up in a month that is already depressing.

One winter afternoon a week before my birthday party I went to a routine medical appointment and agreed to some tests. The sonogram revealed a suspicious growth.

"This mass may well be malignant," the doctor said, and he sent me back to the remedial experience of being a patient in a hospital with instruments pressing against my belly as I stared up at the posters of kittens pinned to the ceiling.

I felt cold, withdrawn, violated. I hid my feelings from the children and—as far as possible—from Byron. I could not imagine throwing a party, but Byron orchestrated a surprise. We went on a road trip, driving around Oregon to look for ghost towns. We saw rolling farmland, tumbleweeds, homesteads falling to pieces in the high desert. We stopped at a largely abandoned town called Friend and walked through the snow to look inside an empty, cold community center sitting open to all passersby, the plain white wooden building covered with chalked graffiti.

The first time I was in the hospital, my friends all came to visit. My parents' friends brought presents. My extended family gave whatever they could: money, rides, anything that was needed. When the second surgery happened, fewer people called. The third, fourth, and fifth surgeries received less attention. By the sixth surgery, my mother was alone watching her only child fade away. It might have been easier to abandon us, but my father just worked harder to pay bills, pumping gas and cleaning toilets, receding into the background.

Some people were too elderly to do much, others were busy with work. The reality of the town did not change just because I had cancer. The only consistent visitor I recall throughout the first few years of hospital stays was the bill collector who had once given my young mother a job as his secretary. He wore a porkpie hat and had cloth handkerchiefs. He brought flowers and patted my mother's arm. The other friends—the people we had gone camping with, the people who had once invited us to every party and celebration—were no longer around.

I was drowning in pain, my mother in sorrow, and it appeared that nobody cared. We were alone together, stranded in the illness, and her only comfort was a pack of Merit cigarettes.

I knew that the abandonment was my fault. I knew that my disease was creepy, that kids are not supposed to get sick and maybe die. I knew exactly how much the whole thing cost, not only the tests and surgeries but also the treats and trips that were meant to distract me. And beyond that, I knew the most frightening cost: the loss of friends.

Waiting for the new test results, I cautiously attempted to tell some of my friends. For the first time, I used direct and clear words to admit that I was scared. Telling the truth felt like a robotic intelligence had taken over my brain and was operating my mouth by remote control. This was an exercise of some sort, a kind of corrective emotional homework. Byron was a stalwart and affectionate companion. Some people offered sympathy and practical assistance with rides and child care. Many other friends acted in a predictable fashion, turning away, unable to hear what I was saying, unwilling to offer help. One woman broke off our friendship abruptly; she said that I was being selfish, asking for too much, even though I hadn't asked for anything at all.

I didn't understand why people I cared about were responding in such different ways. Byron said, "It isn't about you, it's about whatever is going on in their minds, and that isn't something you can predict."

"That doesn't really help me though. If I want to talk about this stuff, what can I do to get through to people?"

Byron laughed and said, "You always talk about medical problems in a flat and disconnected way. If you really want them to understand, you will have to cry."

Weeks passed and a series of tests turned out badly. I tried to ride my bicycle but my mind filled with an almost feral desire to sort through the house and put everything in order. One day I was sifting through more boxes and clothes in the basement and waiting for a chorus friend named Stevie to visit. Instead, Marisa called to say that there had been an accident. Stevie had been riding her bicycle and was hit by a car, run over, and dragged for more than a block.

Dozens of our friends camped in the intensive care visitors' lounge for days at a time, talking to Stevie's parents and rendering aid in some practical fashion. I paced the hallway, walking around a square of brown linoleum that did not match the larger pattern of linoleum in the hallway. The hospital itself was such a painful experience for me that I rarely took my turn to go in and see a mangled young friend. I couldn't handle the smell of the place, the uniforms, the routines. I walked back and forth in the corridor, putting my feet precisely on the brown squares.

When I go to the doctor, I am patient in a literal sense: my heart rate slows down, my blood pressure is unnaturally low. To my profound surprise, I had the opposite reaction when visiting Stevie. I panicked and could barely stand the institutional surroundings long enough to say hello. Watching a dexterous young person suffer was a fresh daily horror. I said to Byron in frustration, "It would be easier not to care about anyone."

The ability to maintain a pristine, steady calm during crisis had always come to my aid in the past. When my aunt was in the final stages of cancer I went to visit, let her hold my baby son, and enjoyed the last opportunity to talk with her. When my grandfather died I was able to efficiently help the children understand what was happening and speak at the funeral. When my grandmother was in hospice I helped tend to her at the end, listening to her chest rattle, watching her face as she died. The grief was not incapacitating until after she closed her eyes for the final time.

It was different with Stevie because she was so young. Standing outside the room and looking through the open door at her closed eyes, at her hair matted with sweat, I may not have known what she was feeling, but I had an approximate idea of what she faced. The process played through my mind like a slide show: the surgeries and treatments, bills and lawsuits, dependence on unwanted help; the life-altering decisions based on the hunch of whichever expert is in front of you; the slow tortuous path to recovery, losing friends, compromising ideals, becoming an observer in your own life. It was a terrible injustice that she should have to go through the experience, that she would learn these secrets.

I could not talk to my friends, could not sit with them in the lounge, but one evening a group found me in the hallway. They clustered close to ask my advice on a point of etiquette. Stevie had ordered everyone to leave the room, and they wondered if they should ignore the request and insist that she accept their help.

"You have to do what she wants or you aren't helping at all," I said, voice cracking. It felt like the room was tilting. I turned and walked down the corridor, brushing tears away with the back of my hand.

I thought they were sticking around because this was a singular crisis, that most of them would disappear if Stevie needed any kind of long-term convalescence. I felt queasy with the instinct that few of these people would have showed up to help me if I needed assistance. But those ideas suddenly appeared false and juvenile; I wasn't thinking about these people, or even Stevie. I was thinking about myself, and the past.

Every second of sadness for Stevie was multiplied by the knowledge that I had been arrogant in judging the people who left me alone during my illnesses. I never understood what it must have been like for them, how painful and frightening it is to watch a young person suffer.

Thinking about the earnest, sweet friends in the visitor's lounge, I knew that I was wrong, that many of them would have given whatever aid was needed. But there was something else, a deeper truth: If they had tried to help me, *I would have sent them away.* The real pathology at the center of my life was not cancer; it was the fact that I refused to let anyone see me as weak.

Stevie's parents had flown in from New York. They were staying in a hotel, didn't know the town, and were struggling to care for a grown-up daughter without treating her like a little child. I gave Stevie's mom a ride back to the hotel, and as I listened to her talk about the doctors and treatments, I was mortified by the glimpse of what my own mother must have gone through.

My mother was young and strong when she gave birth to a baby damaged in unknown ways. The dysfunction of that fragile little body was not her fault, though it was also not part of the plan. She deserved better; and she could have been excused for hating the child who robbed her of youth, innocence, and hope, requiring ever higher investments of time and money. But she held me in her arms and danced across the floor, singing lullabies to soothe my wails. She forced the doctors to pay attention, listen, and save her saturnine little daughter. My mother gave me everything, more than she could afford, more than I deserved.

Growing up I often wondered if I had ruined her life, if she regretted her decision to become a mother. In that moment in the car with Stevie's mom, it occurred to me that the answer to both questions was probably *no*. My mother appreciates me for who I am, entire and whole. My mother loves me in the present tense, the way I love my children no matter what happens. If my mother had been sitting in the car with us, she would have said, "Stop being so morbid and go help your friend."

I made arrangements for the children to stay with their friends after school, set aside my various work projects, and spent as much time at the hospital as possible, ignoring the clawing revulsion I felt in the place. I was in the room the afternoon Stevie went down to surgery. I went through the motions of helping her parents, of changing the washcloth on her forehead, not knowing if she would live through the surgery or, if she survived, whether she would ever walk again. When the orderlies came to wheel her away I whispered in her ear that she was brave and strong and that she would be fine. *Fine.*

Stevie was in the same hospital as my oncologist. Waiting in the doctor's office for an appointment I noticed that my underskirt was disintegrating, the old threads dissolving, the layers of lace and tulle falling apart. Worse yet, I became convinced that it smelled of decay, of the phantom blood of previous owners. The slip was fifty years old.

I looked up and saw that the cupboards containing speculums and gowns were capped with seasonal storage: a plastic pumpkin, a basket with a witch's head, arms embracing the orange-painted wicker. One box had *Syringe Syringe* crossed out with a blue marker and *Halloween! Halloween!* written over it in girlish hand. There was a fake Christmas tree with ornaments affixed to its limbs in its original retail package, resting next to fake Styrofoam presents wrapped in cheery paper. I wondered if people sitting in the

waiting room during the holidays expecting to hear a death sen-
tence were comforted by the seasonal decor.

The oncologist was my age, not a stern old man. He seemed
hyperactive, dazzling, in a lab coat embroidered with his name in
cursive. He knew from my questions that I was in contact with the
people doing research on my disease and seemed relieved by the
fact that I knew more about the particulars of my rare disorder
than he did.

The doctor sat sideways on his swiveling stool, head cocked
and staring at an empty corner of the room. He asked what I
wanted to do about the new test results. We both knew that
exploratory surgery was indicated.

"I want to be healthy, even if I'm just pretending," I replied.

We stared at each other for a long tense moment. Then the
doctor looked down at my chart, shrugged, and said that I could
proceed.

No referral? No lab tests? No surgery, no *cancer*?

I laughed out loud and jumped down from the exam table, a
corner of my petticoat snagging, the layers ripping apart.

scrapbook

From my position in bed, I looked out the window at the lights of Seattle and small fragments of memory flitted through my mind again: the grim, dirty hospital on Beacon Hill and radiation served in a paper cup; the warm, blue hospital on First Hill and an allergic reaction to pain medicine. Doctors pressing forward, always too close.

Still quivering from the morphine, without anything else to dull the pain of the surgery, I put a newspaper over my face and cried.

Byron stroked the portions of my sweaty, matted hair visible above the paper and consoled me the best he could. "It's OK to be scared, Bee," he told me. "You don't have to be so brave."

But the new wounds hurt when I cried, so I had to stop and go back to contemplating the view of moonlight on the water and

the impression of the mountains in the distance. I took off my
glasses and the scene settled into an eerie, anonymous splendor.
The view could have been any city, any body of water, any mountain range in the world.

The resident showed up at seven the next morning. She said
that the surgeon had chased something down my bile duct and
after much effort extracted it; not a gallstone, but something else
that could cause trouble. The gallbladder was bound up in scar
tissue, choked and blackened.

"I think that you should stay another night for observation,
but since you are up and walking you are probably stable enough
to go home. Which would you prefer?"

"I want to go home."

The morning was sunny and cold when I was finally
wheeled out of the hospital by an elderly volunteer, a bottle of
unwanted pain pills stuffed in the travel bag on my lap. Byron
was waiting at the curb with the Volvo and he buckled my seat
belt, then we drove up Beacon Hill toward our home. I hadn't
noticed that the muscles in my neck and back were clenched
until they suddenly relaxed as we pulled into the alley to park. I
opened the car door and swung my legs out, then unexpectedly
retched, spitting clots of blood and chunks of bile onto the
gravel next to the rosemary bush.

We both stared down at the gelatinous mess; Byron laughed
and said, "Would you like to go back to the hospital?"

"No, thank you," I replied, and inched my way toward my
own warm bed.

I slept for an entire day, woke up, and threw the pain medication in the garbage. Moving slowly to avoid jostling the new cuts,

I opened the scientific cabinet and rummaged through the bottom shelf until I found my *E.T.* scrapbook.

My house faces east, away from the forest where I grew up. A few blocks up the hill is the hospital where I drank radioactive isotopes. Just down the valley is the mountain where the accident happened. Leaves had fallen from the deciduous trees and I could see snow-covered peaks from the kitchen window. I sat down at the desk and watched the sky change color as night descended, then opened the scrapbook to the pages covered with hospital bracelets, all the surgeries and tests represented on fading plastic bands. I put the new bracelet with the others but didn't glue it down.

The medical charts and X-rays are lost or archived or burned, the bills paid and discarded. Most of the scars have faded. But I have the *E.T.* scrapbook, and I have the worn red plastic-covered pocket calendar my mother kept. Her precisely scripted notes show the appointments and surgeries, and even as each new specialist or treatment is marked it is still hard to believe what the names and times represent. If I press the calendar to my face I can smell the fading blue ink of her ballpoint pen.

My arms are mottled, green and purple, covered with track marks. The backside of my left hand is a solid yellow welt with black stripes, numb but at the same time tender somewhere down deep between ligament and bone. There are five new scars, or what will become scars after the skin knits together and the bloody bandages are peeled aside to remove the stitches.

It is true that my blood and mind contain secrets. The knowledge of hospital corridors and the threat of injury have given me a constant wakeful awareness of danger. The fact that I am alive is a daily revelation, but it is necessary to do more than just survive.

This morning the children crawled in bed with me, stroked my hair, and covered my face with kisses. Byron filled a hot water bottle and tucked it under my feet. There is food in the refrigerator, delivered by friends who have been picking up the children after school.

Other friends have been calling on the telephone to check on my progress. Dozens more will come to the house for a holiday in a few weeks; they say that I will have to let them do all the work. I probably won't tell them if my stomach still hurts, but I will let them take care of me.

Next week I will ride the ferry home to the peninsula. I will sit on a cracked vinyl bench and stare out the window, hoping the clouds clear long enough to reveal Mt. Rainier as it appears to slide away across the horizon. I will take my parents out to dinner; we will talk and laugh and I'll insist on paying the bill.

Before the bruises fade I will start a new project, or plan a trip, or decide to sell everything and move away to a different country. Not to hide from danger, not to deny the truth of my body, but because I want to live as much as possible while I have the time.

Sometimes I feel a powerful nostalgic sadness for all the beauty destroyed in front of me, but I do not have nightmares. If I remember my dreams at all they are in monochromatic hues, visions of friends reunited, the dead and sick restored to at least one moment of joy. I dream of children laughing, first kisses, vast forests, towering mountains, and deep, cold oceans.

ALSO AVAILABLE FROM AKASHIC BOOKS

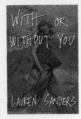

WITH OR WITHOUT YOU
by Lauren Sanders
$14.95, a Trade Paperback Original, ISBN: 1-888451-69-6, 280 pages

"I hate the term poetic, but Lauren Sanders' writing has such a slick mean surface and her subject is such a truly bad girl, a murderer. I mean, so that *poetic* suits *With or Without You* just fine. It's a hot *poetic* book I wouldn't kick out of bed."

—Eileen Myles, author of *Cool for You* and *Chelsea Girls*

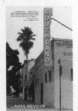

SOUTHLAND
by Nina Revoyr
$15.95, a Trade Paperback Original, ISBN: 1-888451-41-6, 348 pages

Winner of a Lambda Literary Award and a Ferro-Grumley Award
"What makes a book like *Southland* resonate is that it merges elements of literature and social history with the propulsive drive of a mystery, while evoking Southern California as a character, a key player in the tale. Such aesthetics have motivated other Southland writers, most notably Walter Mosley." —*Los Angeles Times*

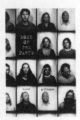

SOME OF THE PARTS
by T Cooper
$14.95, a Trade Paperback Original, ISBN: 1-888451-36-X, 264 pages

A Barnes & Noble Discover Great New Writers Program selection
The novel that's changing the way we define "family." The Osbournes, Sopranos, and Eminem are only "some of the parts" that make up the whole story of the new American family.

"A wholly original novel that's both discomforting and compelling to read . . . "

—*San Francisco Chronicle*

These books are available at local bookstores.
They can also be purchased online through www.akashicbooks.com.
To order by mail send a check or money order to:

AKASHIC BOOKS
PO BOX 1456, New York, NY 10009
www.akashicbooks.com, akashic7@aol.com

(Prices include shipping. Outside the U.S., add $8 to each book ordered.)

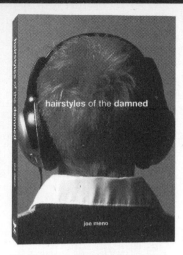
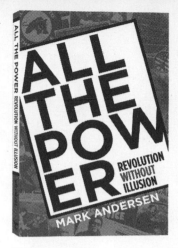
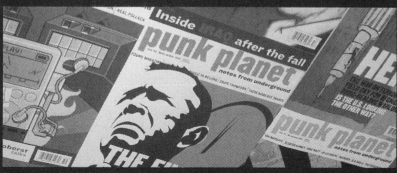

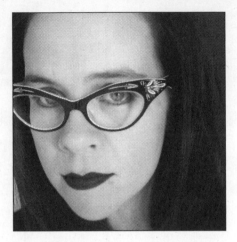

Bee Lavender is a writer, editor, publisher, and activist. After living in the Pacific Northwest for thirty-three years she moved to England, where her office is a canal boat moored on the River Cam. Her previous books include the anthologies *Breeder* (Seal Press, 2001) and *Mamaphonic* (Soft Skull Press, 2004). More information about Bee is available on her website, www.foment.net.